healing hashimoto's naturally

healing hashimoto's naturally

*how i used radical tlc
to love my thyroid and my body
back to health...and you can too!*

Jen Wittman, CHHC, AADP

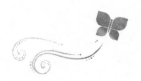

Library of Congress Category-in-Publication Data

Wittman, Jennifer 1975 -

healing hashimoto's naturally: How i used radical tlc to love my thyroid and my body back to health...and you can too! / Jen Wittman

ISBN-13: 978-0-692-34062-2 (The Healthy Plate, LLC)
ISBN-10: 0692340629

Edited by Lacy Boggs
Front Cover Photo by Timothi Jane Graham
Back Cover Photo by Sabrina Hill Weisz
Cover Design by Kevin Plottner
Book Design by Christopher Derrick

DEDICATION

For my husband, Doug, for standing by me through all the ups and downs of illness, every new diet I imposed on the house, every rational and irrational healing modality I tried while you kept our family and household running. I could not have healed without your support.

For Bodhi, who is the inspiration to live vibrantly and healthily every day.

And, for my mom Cindi, dad Chuck and sister, Allison who have all taught and shown me over the years that anything is possible.

CONTENTS

PART 1: CHASING THE BUTTERFLY

PART 2: HEALING THE BUTTERFLY

PART 3: FREEING THE BUTTERFLY

PART 1:

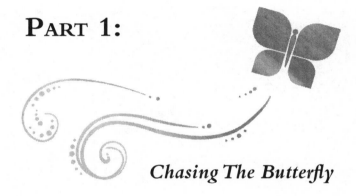

Chasing The Butterfly

CHAPTER 1

Broken Butterfly

"We delight in the beauty of the butterfly,
but rarely admit the changes it has gone through to
achieve that beauty."
- MAYA ANGELOU

I WAS STANDING OUTSIDE OF MYSELF, watching my body lie there, lifeless....unable to lift my head; cloaked in fatigue. Achy in every fiber of my body. I couldn't move. I couldn't get up.

I heard crying from the baby's room. He was ready for mama. He needed me. My help. My love. Some nurturing... but I lacked the energy to give it. As the guilt swelled from my lack of will or want to move, I heard my inner cry. I was so sad.

What had happened to me?

A once vibrant, go-getter, I could hardly manage taking care of my new baby or myself during the day. I didn't even have to go to work. My only job was to take care of the baby and the house but I was failing miserably at both.

My husband was getting annoyed. Every time he came home from a 12 hour day of work to find me on the couch, the house a mess, and me without a smile, was wearing on him. "What was she doing all day?" would be the look across his face.

I remember lying on the bed wanting to crawl out of my skin. As I stared up at the ceiling, waves of panic overtook me... but I wasn't sure why. Before THIS, whatever this was, I could handle any stress...every stress really. Whatever came my way, I was able to deflect, like Wonder Woman with her magic bracelets. Really, stress was no problem. I actually thrived on it. I piled it on, never really feeling it...or so I thought.

Then I had my baby. After that, everything changed. My moods were like a tsunami crashing the shore. At first you're sitting on the beach, enjoying a peaceful sea and in the next moment a tidal wave of anger, sadness, panic would topple me destroying everything in its path. I thought this was just hormones and the intense sleep deprivation of new motherhood but it wasn't. It was something else...something silent and sinister that no one could see.

I suffered alone. I looked normal but wasn't normal...I wasn't even myself. I was a shell. An empty vessel. Nothing.

My Story

My thyroid story starts off like so many others' out there. I spent three years feeling decimated. I had what seemed to be an all-systems breakdown of my body. My body temperature was all over the place. I was having allergic reactions to all sorts of food. I was sleeping too much and then too little; always exhausted. My hair was falling out. My skin was really dry. The list went on and on.

I described the litany of symptoms to a parade of doctors, but every one of them chalked it all up to stress or being a new mom. I insisted that something was off, so the doctors ran some standard blood tests. NORMAL. Ultrasounds were performed. NORMAL. (I started to dread the word NORMAL.)

But I didn't feel normal. I was scared. I didn't know what to do. I hoped they were right, that this was all was due to stress. So I waited and worked on managing my stress. Nothing. No change. I still felt terrible.

"Oh well," I thought. "This must be what motherhood feels like. This must be what my *new normal* is…"

I first realized something wasn't right after I gave birth. I know that having a newborn is exhausting at the best of times, but the level of fatigue I was feeling was off the charts. Everyone was telling me that it was normal, that every new mom was tired. But I could feel in my bones that something wasn't right.

Why is it that all the other new moms I knew were happily

and easily going out into the world with their babies? Yes, they were tired and told tales of long sleepless nights, but they were invigorated by new motherhood, their precious newborns and happy to show off the fruits of their labor. I, on the other hand was not. Getting up and getting ready for the day felt like an insurmountable task. I could literally only put the minimum effort to keeping myself and my beautiful new child alive. I managed to dress myself and feed the baby. That's it. (Luckily, I didn't have to cook for him yet. Thank goodness our bodies supply their first months of nourishment or this kid would have starved.)

While I was pregnant, I started losing more hair in the shower than before. I had heard that during pregnancy my nails and hair would grow stronger. This did not happen to me. I'd asked all my different doctors about it and everyone said that it was due to the hormone shifts in pregnancy; not to worry. Of course, it didn't get better after my son was born, either...

I should have known something was really up when I began noticing deep ridges and what looked like pin holes throughout my nail beds. I already knew a lot about nutrition and physiology and thought this could be a warning that I was malnourished somehow. All the doctors I saw blew it off. They said it was because I was nursing and the baby was getting all that he needed; leaving me a little "depleted." No one suggested that I should support myself through a better diet or supplements or anything else. I was just supposed to blow this off as another "symptom" of new motherhood.

On top of everything else, I was having terrible stomach issues. I ended up in the emergency room twice for intense digestive attacks that turned into panic attacks where I nearly passed out from hyperventilation and severe dehydration. At each hospital visit they "checked" my thyroid and I was in the "normal" ranges. I was fine they said. Probably just the flu or food poisoning.

The girl who disliked hospitals so much that I gave birth at home was begging her husband to take her to the ER, my temperature would swing from one end of the thermometer to the other on a whim, and I was suddenly showing symptoms of being allergic to foods I never had problems with before.

But I was "fine."

I really didn't know what to do or where to turn. I had been to 12 doctors, many of them specialists. I'd had ultrasounds of all my organs, two hospital visits and was even misdiagnosed by a doctor who herself had Hashimoto's disease!

Because all my symptoms were ignored during pregnancy, my son was born with some digestive troubles. We spent his first two years going to doctors, trying to figure it all out. Finally, we were referred to an integrative doctor. After just meeting my husband, son and I and speaking with us for five minutes about my son's health, he asked my husband and son to leave the room. He leaned over his desk and said,

"What's going on with YOU?"

I had never met him before, but he saw my suffering right away. I broke down in tears and described my symptoms to him and he said, "I know what this is but let's give you a blood test to prove it."

Sure enough, he knew what it was. I had Hashimoto's Thyroiditis; an autoimmune disease which affects the thyroid and volleys you back and forth between symptoms of hyperthyroidism and hypothyroidism. What a relief—we finally knew what was going on and it had a name!

But, how did I get here? And what was I going to do about it?

CHAPTER 2

The Slow Road to Sickness

FOR ME, AND FOR MOST PEOPLE, my illness didn't happen all in a moment. It's not as though this butterfly was smashed and broken in a single event, but rather sickened and weakened over a long, long period of time — starting as far back as my childhood.

My grandma cooked; my mom didn't. As long as I can remember, we always had convenience foods in the house. Milano cookies, Chips Ahoy, Spaghetti O's, canned chili, canned vegetables, canned everything and the suite of Hostess goodies. My parents were amazing because of and in spite of that.

My mom was an electrician (totally rad!). There were many days she got us up or left before sunrise to get to work. During our younger years, she fed us a steady diet of "fortified" cereals (read sugar laden), frozen waffles, Pop Tarts. When we were being "healthy," we'd eat cottage cheese and applesauce or a bowl full of blueberries.

My parents did cook, though. I remember them lovingly preparing us Dinty Moore beef stew served with a side of soft

HomePride white bread slathered in Fleischman's margarine. When I think back, the only meal I remember where they actually chopped fresh vegetables was when they took out the ever popular taco kit with the crunchy tacos shells, taco sauce and spice mixture packet. For that meal, they'd chop lettuce, tomatoes and bring out the ol' shredded cheese. It was probably the healthiest meal we ate during that era.

The thing is...they didn't know any better. While my mom and dad were raised on whole foods and my grandmothers were both great cooks, my parents became parents during the age of the convenience foods movement (1970s and 1980s). Where, they were taught by the food companies and federally subsidized food industry that convenience products are better than real food – fortified with extra goodies and healthy for you and your family.

That myth got handed down. I know my parents thought that what they were doing was the right thing for us all. This was the generation of two working parents. No one was home to prepare a fresh home cooked meal every night. There was nothing special about me or my family. This was the story in my friends' homes as well. And as a latch-key kid, I loved the independence that came with taking care of myself and my sister for a few hours as well as feeding myself from an array of goodies like Twinkies and Ding Dongs. I also felt very empowered when I'd snack on a margarined, cheese-filled omelet that I made on the stovetop myself.

Following the breadcrumbs – how my diet made me sick

My parents weren't alone. If you grew up in the 70s or 80s (or had kids during that time), the media was full of messages telling us that factory food was better for us than anything as mundane as an apple or a carrot.

As far back as the early 19th century, at the beginning of the Industrial Revolution, factories began to dictate what was good for us. Back then, the problem was with whole wheat flour. When the germ (the brown part of the wheat seed) was left as part of the flour (what we might today call whole wheat flour), the grains would start to go rancid before the factories could get their flour to market. So the factories invented de-germination — removing the germ from the wheat, which contains most of the nutrition — to solve their problem.

And it worked. They started marketing and promoting the new "white" flour as being healthier because it was more pure — when, of course, nothing could be further from the truth.

And so it went. What was good for the factory must be good for the end user as well.

- Chemicals, additives, flavorings and colorings were all created because they were good for the industrialized food system, and then marketed and sold to us as "improvements" on the food we were used to. Lunchables have a shelf-life of *months* because it's good for Oscar Meyer, not because it's good for the kid eating it. (Have you ever looked at the sodium levels in a Lunchable packet? It's astounding! Take a look the next time you're at the grocery.)

• Genetically modified organisms (GMOs) are another example where what's good for the goose — in this case Monsanto and companies like it — isn't necessarily good for the gander. GMOs are most often created so that the crops can be liberally sprayed with pesticides and herbicides, which aren't good for the environment, the workers or the people who end up eating all those chemicals. They're also created so that the companies can patent seeds — and sue farmers who plant them without paying hefty fees.

• Fortified foods also became all the rage — because as nutritionists realized that we were suddenly lacking certain vitamins and minerals in our diet, the industrial food system jumped on the opportunity to make their food "healthier." The problem is that, while you can add all the vitamins and minerals in a carrot to a piece of bread or a vitamin pill, science shows us that it doesn't necessarily have the same benefits as eating the carrot. All it does is trick us into believing we're eating healthfully.

The American government wasn't blameless in this, either. When the first nutrition guidelines and the familiar food pyramid were released, good nutrition wasn't the guiding force behind them: food lobbies were.

The Secretary of Agriculture gave prominent placement to

grains (suggesting 6 to 11 servings a day!) and dairy because they were powerful lobbies in Washington, not because they were nutritionally more important than other food groups.

The government also espoused the low fat craze that conquered the nation in the 70s, 80s and 90's, which was based on faulty science, but once the government puts its stamp on something it becomes, as it were, law.

So there I was, eating Dinty Moore Beef stew (about one step up from dog chow), Swanson's TV dinners, Pop Tarts, Gatorade, Hostess cakes, Toaster Strudels, Pizza Rolls, and Pepsi — a cornucopia of chemicals and "food-like substances" with hardly a real fruit or vegetable in sight.

PLUS, we were microwaving everything — in plastic containers, no less. Microwaving has been proven to change the nutrients in foods, and the heating process leaches chemicals out of the plastics and into the food. If you only take one thing away from this book, stop microwaving your food (especially in plastic)!

I grew up bombarded with chemicals from my food and drinks, getting very little in the way of whole nutrition, and training my tastebuds only to recognize the overly sweet, salty, fatty tastes a slew of corporations wanted me to like.

It was a recipe for disaster.

Give Yourself Some TLC:

What is your food history? Describe your relationship with food as a child. Did you have enough? Did you eat too much? Good food? Fast food? Did food equate to love in your family? You can download a FREE digital journal at YourBestThyroidLife.com/journal to record your thoughts and memories.

A warning in 8th grade

I spent my youth so hopped up on sugar, I didn't realize my body didn't know what to do with itself. Although my parents were awesome at making us play outside and getting involved in physical activity, my body always felt weak and like it didn't have the energy to really move. I was thin but not a fit person growing up.

One day in 8th grade, my friend's dad who was a heart doctor, observed my behavior: I was manic from all the sugar, unwilling/unable to be that intensely physical to burn it off, and then, of course, crashed. And he looked at me and warned me, "You have symptoms now of someone who will have heart problems when you're older."

Of course, in the 80s, an adult just said stuff like that to you but didn't sit down to further explain it or say what I could do to fix it. He just issued a warning that lived in the back of my head for 3½ decades that I had no understanding of or what to do about it. And, I was only 13 so who cared?

Turns out, I should have. He was spotting early on that my unhealthy habits could add up to something much bigger than a sugar crash in the long run.

Give Yourself Some TLC:

What is your earliest memory of realizing something might be wrong with your health or lifestyle? How did that moment affect you?

College: My first glimpse into "Radical" forms of eating

College is usually when kids get their first taste of being totally in control of their food. On a steady course of doughy Mad Mushroom cheese sticks, midnight beers and Taco Bell, I ended up gaining the Freshman 15. My friends and I would spend hours sitting on the dorm room floor, grabbing and shoving anything cheesy and doughy into our faces.

But after gorging themselves, a few of the girls would mention this thing called a "salad" that I was not familiar with. Apparently, they felt like they needed one of these "salads" to make them feel better. (As I didn't have the taste buds for salad, I wasn't really down with the whole fresh veggies thing.) Some of these girls even mentioned going to an Indian restaurant or vegetarian restaurant in place of eating pizza (a-gain) some nights. This seemed a ludicrous suggestion. Who would eat food like that - fresh food with flavor? Gross.

I merely noted that there were other foods out in the world and was firmly planted in the idea that I wasn't interested in any of that.

By my sophomore year (probably because we'd all gained a fair amount of weight the year before) I noticed that some girls were going to the gym and felt the need to exercise. I really didn't understand that. I thought, "Are these girls so insecure that they have to go to the gym to completely sculpt their bodies?"

It was the same type of girl too - we'll call her a Real Housewife of College.

I thought that the gym sounded like torture and was a completely vain thing to do. It was for a girl who didn't know how to use her brain, who just wanted to look pretty so she could get her M.R.S. degree.

I just stopped eating cheese sticks and beer at midnight and lost the weight. It didn't even occur to me that going to the gym would make me fitter and even feel better. I didn't consider that it would help my overall health. I pretty much vowed to never go to the gym — that was for other people; not for me.

Give Yourself Some TLC:

How did your relationship to food and health change when you were a young adult, on your own for the first time?

California: Life in the palm trees

When I first moved to Los Angeles, shortly after college, my diet still primarily consisted of Gatorade, Hostess Ding Dongs, Taco Bell and any fried or battered bar food. This made grocery shopping pretty uninteresting – throwing boxes of processed and prepackaged foods into the cart, nary a piece of lettuce in sight.

But within the first few weeks of my time here, I began to witness a phenomenon at the grocery. People were putting fruits and vegetables in their carts. They were also walking around in workout clothes. They appeared to be at the grocery store after having gone to something called "a gym." And, they all seemed pretty chipper.

Young or old, I noticed fit, healthy looking people, walking around the grocery store, putting food from the produce section into their carts. This was also the time when fresh, bottled smoothies, Robeks and Jamba Juice were all the rage. People would discuss the best, most power-packed combinations of fruits, veggies and powders for their drinks. I wondered, "What's so wrong with this simple, delicious Gatorade? After all, it's thirst aid "for that deep down body thirst."

Well, there must be something in the water in California, because I finally joined a gym for the very first time in 1999. I only succumbed to it because my company was paying for gym memberships...so I thought, why not? Apparently, my company believed that going to the gym would make healthier, happier employees.

About a week into this new way of life, I realized that I had missed the boat for years. I felt great. This changed the way I looked at health and fitness forever. I had a new respect for my body... but, I was still fueling that amazing body with total crap.

I was also living a high stress life and living near the airport where I breathed in jet fuel for years. While I was fortunate enough to live only a block from the beach at the time (that was pre-2005 real estate bubble), my little beach town was right next to LAX.

L.A. itself is a beautifully intoxicating, yet toxic, city whether it be the smog, the stress or the jet fuel. I essentially breathed in mercury laden jet fuel for 13 years.

Mercury, along with other heavy metals, can interfere with enzyme production - including the enzymes that tell the thyroid to make the T3 and T4 thyroid hormones it's supposed to make. So, mercury from the environment, ingested from large fish, or even vapors off-gassing from old mercury fillings in your mouth can have a serious effect on your thyroid.

During that time I was also faced with the possible diagnosis of cervical cancer - that scared the crap out of me, and my best friend from culinary school, Debbie, gave me a book called, "Healing Foods." It changed the way I thought about food forever.

I started using food as a way to heal my body and eliminate symptoms. Instead of reaching for the Tums, the aspirin, a sleeping aid, I looked to food for some relief. This was a step in the right direction. However, because I was young and healthy-ish, I didn't realize there was still something lurking in the background but that was yet to come.

Give Yourself Some TLC:

How do you medicate yourself? Make a list of everything from aspirin to allergy medication to food and alcohol or prescription (or even recreational) drugs. If you are having to medicate at least one issue a day, there may be something else going on.

The Transition: The 7-year itch

You've probably heard of the idea of the "seven-year-itch," but did you know there's science that backs it up? Most of the cells in your body die off and regenerate, and there's a theory that it takes about 7 years for those cells to completely replace themselves. You may have heard the theory that your taste buds change every 7 years - it's the same idea.

But is it possible that your mind - your hopes, dreams, aspirations - change, too?

For 7 years while my husband and I lived and worked in L.A., I saved money to be able to live my dream of cooking and living in Italy. I could sense that my body needed a change. I knew I needed to slow down but wasn't sure how to do that in Los Angeles. The city is electric and there are so many wonderful things to do, to see, to be, that it's very hard to unplug there...and this was even the time *before* cell phones were commonplace!

We decided that moving to Italy would be that change. So, after 7 years in L.A., we packed it up to head to Italy ... but first we needed to make a stop home.

While we were in Indiana for the summer, my husband noticed that his parents were complaining of ill-health a lot. So, he went to the bookstore (yes, we had those back then!) and found a book he wanted to share with them called, "Never Be Sick Again." He wanted to read through it before he handed it off to them to make sure it was a fit. What he read was eye-opening and he encouraged me to read it too....and I did. It blew me away.

It was the first time I had an understanding of the toxic burden on our bodies from air pollution, chemicals in food and body products and hyper-scheduled living. Boing! Can you see how big my eyes are right now? I couldn't believe it!

It seemed like a perfect transition to the next phase of our lives: slower living and cleaner eating in Italy.

Give Yourself Some TLC:

What environmental factors may be contributing to your health? How many beauty products, cleaning products, chemical food additives, etc. do you come in contact with each day? Do you live in the city? Near a freeway? Near an airport? Near an industrial area? List as many factors as you can think of.

CHAPTER 3

The Great Epiphany

THE ITALIAN LIFESTYLE, while not perfect, turns our currently crazed culture on it's head — in a good way! In Italy, you are not expected to rush around, in fact, that's frowned upon. My days in Italy consisted of a light, traditional Italian breakfast, followed by work or school, followed by a few hours off for lunch to enjoy my meal and catch up with friends. Then, back to work we'd go (usually on foot) and then to a very simple but delicious dinner and post dinner stroll around the town. No rush, no fuss.

People don't dread running into friends or family on the street; knowing they not only have the time, but it's perfectly acceptable to pause and chat with a friend... Being a few minutes late to something doesn't ruffle any feathers. In the US, time is a precious commodity; never feeling like we have enough of it. There, LIFE is the precious commodity and there is always time to do, explore or visit without the pressure of hyper-scheduled living.

One major difference I noticed immediately was Italians don't ask you what you "do" for a living. They don't care. Your career doesn't define who you are or your status. What they care more about is family, food, beauty and fun. They want to discuss your latest adventure, music, food, intellectual ideas. And, the TV is so bad there, people don't need to or even want to spend hours in front of it!

Italians also don't spend hours over the stove like some people assume. Instead, they create simple, delicious meals from the best ingredients. When you go to a grocery store in Italy, you are not bombarded with aisle after aisle of processed, chemical-laden foods; instead, the markets are filled with fresh fruits, vegetables and meats, etc. Many meals are made easily from a few simple, whole food ingredients and are full of flavor.

We ate prosciutto, cheese, bread, yogurt, eggs, wine, espresso, olives, artichokes, eggplant & fruit, Kinder chocolate, gelato. We shopped daily and could only buy what we could carry up 104 stairs. Hey – what more do you need when you're in Italy?

When we lived in Italy, my day started off by walking down those 104 stairs to the neighborhood "bar" (the place where you get breakfast), where I'd order a cappuccino and a pastry at the counter every single day. At lunch time, I would select some of the finest cheese, meat and olives I could afford and buy a loaf of fresh baked bread. I'd end at dinner at a little trattoria enjoying what Italy is world-famous for—fresh, local meats, vegetables, risottos, perfect pizzas or a rich, delicious, pasta dish that was out of this world. We'd often end dinner with a doughy, sweet treat and an espresso or digestivo.

Italians take time to stop and smell the roses. They appreciate good music, their friends and family, and find beauty in many things. They cherish slowing down and really experiencing life. In the afternoons, businesses are closed for a couple of hours so people can eat a nutritious lunch and spend time with their families.

Before or after dinner, it's common to see people taking a *passeggiata* or little, a leisurely walk around the neighborhood greeting friends or walking off a meal. Now, that seems crazy in our hustle/bustle culture but there are ways to steal away little leisurely moments throughout the day so you can reconnect and process thoughts and your food.

Give Yourself Some TLC:

When do you feel you were living your best, most authentic life? Why? What made it so amazing? What steps have you already taken toward living the life you want? Make a big TA-DA list to celebrate!

Hitting the wall, literally:
a recipe for disease

My adventure in Italy was the best in my life. I finally learned what truly fulfilling, healthy, happy life could look and feel like.

Living *la dolce vita* had put me on the right track to healing the butterfly, my body, myself. I thought I had it figured out when I moved back to the States...but I wasn't prepared for what was about to hit me.

It was a Saturday morning. I was happy, I was young, and I was about to do my favorite thing – spend an endless amount of time perusing the aisles of Trader Joe's. The following day would be Mother's Day and my husband and I were going to prepare a special brunch for my mom at her house. It was one of the only times I actually lived in Indianapolis in my adult life and I was excited to spend Mother's Day with my mom in person.

It was an average sort of morning. We had just dropped my car off at the shop for repairs. Then we were going to ride together to the store to prepare for our big feast. Menu and grocery list in hand, we took off happily — not realizing that within 10 minutes, our lives would be forever changed.

We were riding in my husband's Volvo station wagon...a car I took a lot of pleasure in making fun of. It was a total soccer mom car, but we were yet to be parents. I looked for opportunities to tease him about the car and actually loathed driving around in it. I mean, it was a way nicer car than my Civic but my Civic was sporty and a stick shift and something that young people drive. Anyway, I jumped into his mom-mobile and off we went on I-465 northbound to the only Trader Joe's in the area.

The highway was relatively empty except for us and a semi-truck. We were about a ½ mile away from our exit and decided to move into the right lane so we could exit. It was just starting to sprinkle...really it was that spittle rain that's hard to wipe off your windshield but wet enough to make it hard to see. Anyway, we moved over into the right lane alongside this semi-truck.

As we approached the exit, we were a tad ahead of the semi. We were chatting away, enjoying our tea and our time together (oh, the free time of being a couple without children!) when all of a sudden, I saw the front of the truck veering into our lane.

I couldn't think fast enough. Instead of clearly instructing my husband as to what to do, I yelled, "Watch out! Watch out! Watch out!" as the semi-truck barreled into the left back bumper of our car.

The initial impact was jarring, forceful. For a second, I didn't realize what was happening. Because of the slick pavement, we were pushed forward in front of the truck now….spinning around and around across four lanes of traffic. Time slowed down. I was able to consciously look at my husband and see the oncoming cars.

I remember thinking, "We're gonna get hit by another car" and then the thought, "I-can't-believe-THIS-is-how-I'm-going-to-die." Just as that thought entered my head, I could see myself dead across the divider on the other side of the highway...I was taken out of that by the sound of my husband yelling.

"Hold on!"

At that moment, the car straightened out and I felt it dip down and head directly for the cement highway divider.

I was about to hit the wall, literally.

As we were violently propelled forward, I felt something push me back into my seat...and then I smelled smoke. I looked up, dazed. Smoke was filling the cabin of the car.

All I could think was that the car was going to explode.

I jumped out of the car and stumbled onto the highway. I grabbed the phone...my only thought was I needed my mom. I must call my mom.

When you're in an accident like that, your brain and body go into survival mode. You can't think straight. You're not even aware of what's happened to you. So much adrenaline is coursing through your body that you don't realize....you've been injured or how severely.

Within days, the full magnitude of the accident began to reveal itself. At age 31, I had a debilitating hip injury, my skeleton on the right side was completely out of alignment and the muscles couldn't hold it all together correctly. I had PTSD and a mild traumatic brain injury.

Even suffering from just one of those would be challenging,

but dealing with all of that propelled me into the abyss of depression and an era of non-stop fight or flight living.

Stress: can't live with it...

Adding a little insult to injury, the truck company's insurance company decided they didn't want to pay for our medical bills, even though their driver admitted being at fault. He admitted to never having used his sideview mirrors and he admitted to driving for more than 24 hours (a complete legal no-no). The company records even showed that this driver had several safety violations and had failed many safety exams but they were unwilling to pay for the damage to our bodies and lives.

Let's take a second to really look at that damage too. As I mentioned, I suffered a debilitating hip injury, PTSD and a brain injury. I had to go on disability because I couldn't drive to my office or perform the tasks of my job as a chef and caterer. I couldn't dance, do any physical activities I used to do (I'm talking ANY of them) and I was having neurological problems.

The truck hit us two weeks before we were moving back to California. I had just received my highest paying job offer ever...one that was a game changer and completely deserved after an already 10 year career in my industry. But now I couldn't take the job. I couldn't even move to California with my husband. He had to leave for California without me and start his job while I moved back in with my mom and stepdad so I could be cared for until I healed enough that I could make the trip across the country.

All of this happened, and instead of the truck company paying for the damage they caused, they put us on trial as two people trying to game the system....trying to take advantage of the poor, sweet truck company. They hired a P.I. to follow us in California. They tried to make us out to be these sly kids trying to scam them... The truck company that put an unsafe driver on the road, pressured him to drive more than the allowable hours and who hit us because of his negligence.

Now, if you haven't lived in California before, you might not know how crazy expensive it is here. Our small two bedroom apartment cost more in rent than my mom's large house on a nice parcel of land in Indiana. The truck company was trying to make it seem like we were rich and out to screw them. They dug up anything they could from our past to twist around and try to make their case. They even had an "independent" medical examiner write a report that said I had PTSD from the events of 9/11 and not from the accident!

So, while I was trying to heal my body and mind from all of this, my husband and I were under fire and being followed for 5 years. And, if you've ever been involved in a lawsuit before, you understand how the laws often protect the big guy and not the little people.

Our attorney let us know we were being followed and encouraged us not to even smile when we were outside. I was told never to pick up my new baby son in public because the PI would get a picture of that and use it to "prove" I didn't actually have a hip injury. Now you tell me: what mother, regardless of pain, suffering or a terrible injury wouldn't pick up her child or hold her infant in public, especially when that baby needed her?

And even worse, I lost my career and by proxy, my identity as a chef — the one thing I had worked toward my entire adult life. So there I was, an injured person, unable to work, unable to be intimate with my husband, unable to care for my newborn and unable to be myself in public because the truck company didn't want to pay the medical bills for injuries they'd caused. Can you say STRESS?

That's when I started to feel worthless. Never before had I experienced that. I had always had an abundance of self-love and self-worth. Did I mention my parents were awesome? To feel worthless and depressed was something new to me...and it felt like something that would never change. Who was I now?

Emotional Eating

You can imagine that while I was going through that, I wasn't reaching for an apple to comfort my soul. No, I was suppressing my pain with pastries, donuts, coffee, pasta, snack foods, the works! Although I emotionally felt better as I ate these foods (temporarily), I started to feel sicker and sicker and didn't know why. My body seemed to crave these foods and I believed that following my body's messages were the most important thing I could do at the time. And the message was to Eat. More. Cake.

Of course, that was the last thing I needed. Just like my friend's father told me in the 8th grade, sugar wasn't doing my body any favors. My blood sugar was wildly out of whack, fueling my emotional roller coaster, and the constant stress of too much sugar was a strong set-up for insulin resistance.

Baby Steps

Having a baby was the best and worst thing that ever happened to me. It was the best because my husband and I created the most precious little creature/little rascal in the world. Our hearts exploded the day he was born and it has been and will continue to be the most important experience in my life.

But, having a baby sent me on a journey I wasn't expecting... something I never asked for, something I would never wish on my worst enemy. Having a baby was the tipping point and the reason why Hashimoto's was able to take hold.

The hormonal shifts during pregnancy make many women ripe for Hashimoto's and other thyroid challenges.

When I look back at my life so far, the clues that I was on the wrong path and how to get on the right path were right in front of my face all along....but just like most people, I'm human and hindsight is 20/20. I ignored the warnings, didn't pay attention to the signs. My life's story basically took me on a journey to illness, to a personal hell, to a breaking point - and then on a life-long passion for health and healing.

Give Yourself Some TLC:

Which of the common risk factors for Hashimoto's do you have? Could you be suffering from Hashimoto's? Look back on all your answers so far and take this quiz at **www.freethyroidquiz.com** to find out.

PART 2:

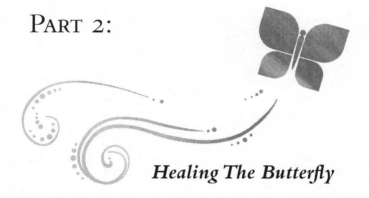

Healing The Butterfly

CHAPTER 4

Learning to Live — and Love — Again

AT MY LOWEST POINT, it wasn't just me who was suffering from my Hashimoto's disease; my infant son and my marriage were suffering in a big way as well. My husband and I had some very raw talks in which we admitted how we were both experiencing the thyroid disease that had befallen me—and how it was tearing our family life and love apart.

My husband missed his friend and partner-in-crime...the girl who kept him in hijinks, hilarity, love and affection. The adventurous girl who was always out for exploration and new journeys.

Now, he came home to a wife who was unable to work, could hardly move herself off the couch and did absolutely no house work. Someone who could only give her wee bit of energy to their newborn but had none leftover for him or anyone else.

I was a shadow of myself....almost a ghost of a person... and the worst part was that I looked "fine." From the outside, I looked like a healthy new mom while inside everything was falling apart...my body was attacking me.

Finally, we had both had enough. We'd had enough of my suffering and the neglect to the rest of our life together. After expressing tough feelings, we committed to beating thyroid disease together. As a force, we were able to support each other so I could reverse thyroid disease.

I could never have healed if I hadn't reached out for help and enlisted my friends and family in the process. Once I was honest with them and asked for their help, I had the support I needed so that I could reduce stress, have time to do things that would be healing to my mind, nervous system and organs and I was quickly able to reverse disease.

But the truth is that I couldn't have taken that all-important step of asking for help if I hadn't been able to dig deep and find enough love *for myself* to want to get better.

As it turns out, Hashimoto's disease and depression, anxiety, and panic attacks go hand-in-hand. The adrenals, thyroid and our gut are inextricably linked. So it's a chicken and egg scenario as to whether a malfunctioning thyroid affects your adrenals or if your adrenals are taxed and that affects your thyroid.

It also creates a perfect recipe for depression: Your hormones are out of whack, your body is malfunctioning on a very basic level, yet no one can see any sign of injury or pain.

When you're in that dark place, it's hard to imagine a way out. But I can tell you from experience that the only way out, the only way back to health, is through love.

Love is what finally brought me back from the brink and allowed me to heal and reverse the symptoms of my disease.

- The love of my husband and my family and friends supported me, held me up when I needed it, and assured me that even though I was the only one who could make the journey back to health, I wasn't alone.

- My love for my son and husband lit a fire in me to want me to be better for them. I desperately wanted to be the mother and wife they needed, wanted, and deserved.

- But most of all, I had to uncover the love for *myself* that was the ultimate drive I needed to undertake a journey back to health.

Giving myself a little TLC.

"How much we know and understand ourselves is critically important, but there is something that is even more essential to living a wholehearted life: <u>loving</u> ourselves."
– BRÉNE BROWN

This is what I call the caterpillar stage of the healing process (which you'll learn about more in the next chapter). It happens when you've decided you're ready for a change and you're willing to take the steps to nourish yourself back to health.

Of course, that's easy for me to say now, but in the beginning, the enormity of the lifestyle changes I was facing was overwhelming. My research was showing me to give up foods I had eaten my entire life, habits that had shaped the very core of my personality — things I thought made me, *me*.

I was a chef, for God's sake! I grew up Midwestern where bread and cheese are major food groups! And my biggest dream in life was to be an Italian transplant — eating any delicious ingredient I want (healthy or not) like pizza and pastry every day of the week. I wanted no food groups off the table.

How could I give those things up without losing myself in the process?

Getting rid of the stress in my life was another major hurdle. As enticing as it sounded to have someone else doing the laundry or unloading the dishwasher, the thought of actually asking for help (and thereby admitting that I wasn't actually Wonder Woman) was scary.

My husband already knew I was a wreck, but what would my friends say if I asked them to watch my son once in a while? What would people think of me if I hired a housekeeper?

I won't lie to you. I was resistant to the idea of all of these changes at the beginning. Then I thought maybe I could try it for a while — almost just to prove to myself that it wouldn't make me any better! Then I entertained the idea that after I "fixed" myself, I could go back to my old ways.

That was over three years ago, and I can honestly say I've never looked back.

It takes a lot of courage to make these kinds of changes. To ask for the help you need, you must love yourself more than you love the *image* of yourself being able to "do it all." To make changes when you don't know what the outcome will be requires courage and a conviction that you will keep trying things until you find what works best for you.

The place to start? Understanding where you're at with your journey. Knowledge is power, so head to **freethyroidquiz.com** and find out where you stand.

The changes I made showed myself I cared, that I was important, that I deserved to heal — and *that* was the most important change of all.

In the midst of this process, I've learned something surprising: disease and healing have one very important thing in common: vulnerability.

When you're sick, you're vulnerable because you have no choice. Your body is doing things, reacting to things that seem beyond your control. You tumble into vulnerability because there is no other way to survive. You must ask for help. You must show "weakness" in front of others. You must succumb to the demands of your physical needs.

Being sick is being vulnerable. You don't know what's going to happen next. You feel like you have to put your trust in others to get through. It's a very scary place for most of us to be.

But the flip side of that is the vulnerability in healing. Unlike sickness, healing (when it comes to Hashimoto's and diseases like it) is a choice. But it's a choice filled with vulnerability. You must be vulnerable enough to ask for *more* help. You must be vulnerable enough to trust the process and yourself. You must push through that intense fear and vulnerability to take the first step and commit to change.

"If I knew for sure it would heal me..."

I have a friend who came to me for help with her son's health. He had a hard time focusing, was hyperactive, hyper-sensitive to stimulation and generally out of sorts. After doing a dietary assessment, it became clear to me that gluten and sugar were his triggers. I encouraged my friend to eliminate gluten from their diet. She wasn't thrilled at the prospect. She said, "If I knew 100% for sure that eliminating gluten would change everything for the better, I'd do it. It's just too overwhelming to make that sort of huge change in our family if there are no guarantees."

I understood where she was coming from. I felt the same way when I learned that eliminating gluten might help me in my healing journey. I DID NOT want to make that change. What if I made that change and it didn't work? Why did I want to torture myself even further?

I realized this was my fear talking and recognized this fear in my friend. Sometimes, changes feel daunting. But what is the alternative? Continuing to suffer because we're unwilling to take a chance on something that could help? We're afraid of trying something new and it failing? THAT is vulnerability right there. Trying something new without the guarantee of success.

Why are we such slaves to foods? Back in the day, people didn't have the luxury of thinking about real food as a choice, a convenience. Food was nourishment, sustenance, survival. It wasn't something focused on, talked about, dissected. Food was just food. You ate the real stuff and didn't eat what made you feel gross. So, why are we so attached to foods that harm us these days? Sweets, processed foods and glutenous gobbledegook?

I'm just as guilty as anyone else. As you've learned from my experience above, I was just as resistant as the next guy. It was only when I made the choice to take a chance and make the change, to show my body the love it needed to heal, to surrender to the healing process that things began to change for me.

I shared my experience with my friend and encouraged her to get vulnerable and make these two important changes for her family. The alternative was watching her son suffer and to continue feeling stressed because of his behavior. What was the harm in giving it a shot, after all?

After our heart to heart, my friend decided to surrender to something new, a different way of doing things that just might make the difference between heartbreak and healing. And, it was a success! By making those simple changes, the life of her family changed forever. Her son was able to focus, do better in school, handle stress easier and be a happy member of the family. Making that change created space for her entire family to thrive!

As that quote from Bréne Brown says, "we can understand ourselves fully, but the key to a wholehearted life is <u>loving</u> ourselves."

The same can be said for healing: You can understand every last thing about your disease, but the only way to live a whole life again is to love yourself enough to make the leap and choose healing.

Give Yourself Some TLC:

Spend some time really exploring any beliefs you have that are standing in the way of healing. Here are just a few of the *many* I've heard working with clients to get you started:

- I can't change the way I eat because my family won't want to eat that way.
- My partner can't help out more at home because he works so much outside the home.
- The house/family would fall apart if I don't manage everything.
- My friends won't understand if I ask for help.
- My boss won't let me change my schedule (even though I haven't asked).
- I don't have time to work out or meditate.
- My mother would be so disappointed in me if she knew I _____

What is your first reaction to each statement? If it rings true for you, explore why and write about it in your journal.

How I learned to fall in love with myself again.

Let me tell you one important thing I learned from being sick: It is *hard* to love yourself when your body isn't doing what you want it to! When you are sick and tired (and tired of being sick and tired!), when it feels like your body has betrayed you, when your weight isn't where you want it to be, when your hair is falling out — it's *really* hard to remember how to love yourself.

But what I had to relearn — and what I would love to help you remember — is that I was still the same person underneath. My mood was wonky, my fingernails were brittle, my stomach was rebelling, but those were all just symptoms.

And we are *not* our symptoms.

Underneath all the trial and tribulation I was going through, I was still the same Jen, and if I could find the strength to love myself, the rest would take care of itself. I was not "my" disease. I would not let thyroid disease define me.

One of the most important changes I had to make was inside my head: my self-talk. It's so easy to fall into the trap of saying, "I can't do that," or focusing on the things we don't like — our self-perceived "flaws."

But that kind of negative self-talk is incredibly damaging. Think of some of the awful things you say to yourself on a daily basis — "I'm too fat," or "I can't do anything any more," or "I look ugly." Would you say any of those things to a 6 year old child? I'm betting you wouldn't!

So why are you saying them to yourself?

Whenever you start on a self-talk rant, remember, there's a 6 year old child that lives in you (in all of us). Aren't you worthy of as much love as she is? (The answer, in case you were wondering, is a resounding YES!)

One way to change this barrage of self-criticism is to focus on the positive. Did you get out of bed today? Way to go! Did you get dressed and take the kids to school? That's a WIN! Did you fix yourself a healthy meal? OMG you're a winner!!!

Sound a little crazy? It's not. Healing is all about baby steps, and every baby step is a win. So acknowledge those wins and celebrate them! Train yourself to be a little more kind and positive, and it will pay big dividends.

Even when you *don't* win, it's important to acknowledge your effort. Let's say you wanted to vacuum the house, but you only made it through one room before you needed to rest. (Happened to me SO MANY times.) Don't berate yourself for not doing the whole house! Instead, acknowledge what you *did* do. "Well, I managed to vacuum one room today, and tomorrow I can do another one."

The other side of this coin is to forgive yourself for any mistakes. Let's face it: some days, you may feel like you absolutely cannot live without that chocolate chip cookie. Here's the secret: If you ate it, it's not the end of the world. Even if you've told yourself you've given up gluten and sugar — and you ate the cookie anyway — don't dwell on the mistake! Forgive yourself and move on. Start over right away at the very next opportunity.

As I continued to grow and heal, I started a self-love practice every single day. Here's what my routine looks like:

- Stress Reduction: 10 minutes for meditation/breathing exercises

- Fitness: 30 minutes for light exercise

- Detox: 30 minutes for a daily Epsom salt bath or sauna

- Self-love: 10 minutes for writing in my journal

- Brain reboot:10 minutes for a walk outside or around the office mid-day

- R & R: 30 minutes for something playful (doing a hobby, horsing around with my son, dancing to my favorite music, watching a funny TV show, trading massages with my honey, something that will make me laugh and smile)

I commit to myself 2 out of 24 hours every day so that I can feel better, have the energy to do all the things I want to do and be the friend, parent, partner, colleague, and daughter I want to be. (I talk about why I chose each of those activities in later chapters.)

You may be thinking that this sounds like a lot, or that it sounds awfully woo-woo that journaling and thinking positively will heal you, but here's the honest truth: Until you make a decision to love yourself, you cannot heal. You are basically telling the universe (and all the people around you) that you aren't worth it, you aren't worthy of feeling better, you don't deserve to be healthy.

And I know that's not true (whether you've figured it out yet or not!).

Give Yourself Some TLC:

Why do you deserve love? Set a timer and free write for 10 minutes about why you deserve to be loved. Don't be surprised if this brings up some powerful emotions! Now ask yourself, how will you start loving yourself back to health?

CHAPTER 5

The Three Phases of Healing

KNOWLEDGE IS POWER, especially when it comes to your body.

Because of a medical system that is sorely lacking in understanding and education of thyroid, autoimmune and inflammatory disorders, it's more important than ever to be educated on the basics of these diseases, the testing that can help you really understand what's going on with your body, and how to address the root causes.

As you probably well know, misdiagnosis is all too common with thyroid, autoimmune and inflammatory disorders—and an accurate diagnosis is the first step in choosing your best treatment on your road to health. The thyroid functions through a complex series of steps, and the process can break down at any one point along the way.

Unfortunately, in our Western medical system, if you go to your doctor with thyroid symptoms, chances are that you'll just be given a prescription for replacement hormones—without ever diagnosing the *cause* of your problems. It's flat out wrong to assume that all thyroid disorders should be treated the same way, but that's the way most doctors treat them.

Even more frustrating, if your lab tests come back "normal" they may not do anything except tell you you're fine!

This chapter will walk you through the rudimentary basics of what your thyroid is, how it is supposed to function, what might be going wrong, and how to diagnose it.

Knowledge is power! So let's get started!

Thyroid Basics

If you're anything like me, you probably never gave a thought to your thyroid until someone suggested it might be to blame for all the symptoms you were having. (Like that song says, "You don't know what you've got 'til it's gone...") I honestly didn't know I had a thyroid until mine stopped working. Well, actually, as I learned over time, my thyroid is functioning, but it was under siege. My body had been mounting an autoimmune attack on my thyroid and I learned everything I could to stop the attack. Here's a brief overview of your thyroid and what you really need to know.

What is your thyroid?

The thyroid is a butterfly-shaped gland located in your throat, right below your Adam's apple. The thyroid makes, stores and releases thyroid hormones (T3 and T4) into your blood. This process affects almost every cell in your body, helping control the body's functions and it has a profound effect on cellular energy and metabolism.

Thyroid imbalances come in two major forms, hyperthyroidism and hypothyroidism. Hypothyroidism is when there is too little thyroid hormone in your blood. This makes your body and its functions sluggish. Hyperthyroidism, on the other hand, is when you have too much thyroid hormone in your blood and everything starts racing.

Hashimoto's thyroiditis is a condition in which your own immune system attacks the thyroid, and often results in hypothyroidism but can volley you back and forth between hypo- and hyperthyroid symptoms. Hashimoto's disease is progressive, and can be difficult to diagnose, as your thyroid levels can start out within the "normal" range but still not be at optimal levels (which I discuss the significance of later). It is only one cause of hypothyroidism, but it is the most common.

How does your thyroid work?

Science is discovering more and more that the systems in our body don't function as separate pieces, but rather all influence one another, and your thyroid is no exception.

The thyroid gland works together with your pituitary gland and hypothalamus to control the amount of thyroid hormone in your body. For some of you, this information will be old hat. But for those just starting out, here's a closer look at how the thyroid works.

The hypothalamus gland sends a message using thyroid releasing hormone (TRH) to your pituitary gland.

1. Your pituitary gland then determines how to stimulate the thyroid by sending thyroid stimulating hormone (TSH).

2. TSH stimulates your thyroid to produce inactive T4 and active T3 (thyroid hormones);

    a. The inactive T4 goes to your liver and intestinal tract to be converted to active T3.

    b. Active T3 goes straight to the bloodstream to be delivered to your cells.

Important Takeaway: Active T3 is the hormone used by our cells to produce energy and protective steroid hormones. Our thyroid only makes 10% of the active T3 we need to function properly. The rest of the Active T3 (the other 90%) is created when T4 gets converted in the liver.

The more I've learned about the thyroid, the more it seems to be in charge of everything that goes on in the body from basic aspects of body function to all the major systems. (It's actually kind of annoying that it's such a big deal!) Every cell in our body has thyroid hormone receptors, and so every system in your body can be affected when your thyroid is off.

To actually help your thyroid remember how to function properly again, you have to address several of those other systems. For instance, thyroid hormones are responsible for many basic functions in the brain, the G.I. tract, the gallbladder and liver, the cardiovascular system, bone and red blood cell metabolism. If your thyroid function is low, you can experience hair loss, weakened bones, depression and infertility. As we all know too well, the thyroid also affects temperature regulation, hormone production and our metabolism. Fat, bald and moody, anyone?

Hashimoto's: the hidden thyroid epidemic

Are your TSH levels in the "normal" range but you're experiencing almost every thyroid symptom under the sun? If so, you're not alone, and you're not crazy!

If you suspect you have a thyroid problem but it's not showing up on the standard panel, it is important you check to see whether an autoimmune condition called Hashimoto's is at play.

I'm finding there is a lot of confusion out there on what hypothyroidism is and how that differs from Hashimoto's (autoimmune) thyroiditis. The crucial difference is in what's affecting your thyroid. With hypothyroidism, your gut, adrenals, stress levels, thyroid hormone conversion problems, and a host of other things could be challenging thyroid function. With Hashimoto's, thyroiditis occurs when the body inadvertently creates antibodies to signal T-cells to attack the thyroid tissue itself. So often, you're thyroid is working "fine" but it is under fire as the body is destroying its own thyroid tissue.

If you have Hashimoto's, you will approach healing a little differently than if you are just dealing with hypothyroidism. In addition to the important dietary and lifestyle changes you can make to support healing your thyroid, with Hashimoto's you have to address the autoimmune response itself. What has a lot of practitioners, doctors, and researchers stumped is that what stops the autoimmune response for some doesn't work for others, but we'll cover the options that have worked for many.

Hashimoto's causes chronic inflammation of the thyroid and is important to get a handle on right away. It is also the #1 cause of hypothyroidism and commonly goes undetected because it's not included in the standard thyroid test panel. Make sure to ask your doctor to test your TPO and TGB antibody levels. It's important to take antibody tests a few times. If you get a single negative result, that doesn't mean you don't have Hashimoto's which is why it is important to test your antibody levels multiple times. Sometimes, the immune system can be so suppressed that antibodies aren't being produced.

There are other thyroid patterns that are important to look into that are not part of standard lab testing. There are some patterns of thyroid imbalance that do not readily show up on standard lab tests. This is why 60–80% of thyroid disorders go undiagnosed or misdiagnosed in the United States every year. These patterns indicate thyroid dysfunction and likely you'll be experiencing symptoms but your doctor will not have the right information to diagnose and treat you effectively. So, it's important that you be on the lookout for the following patterns:

Under-conversion of T4 to T3

As the inactive thyroid hormone, T4 must be converted to T3 before it can be used by your body, but more than 90% of what your body makes for itself is T4.

If you have inflammation and elevated cortisol levels, it can damage your body's ability to convert T4 to T3. If this is what is happening in your body, you'll have hypothyroid symptoms, but your TSH and T4 levels will be normal. To diagnose this dysfunction, have your T3 tested, and it should show as low.

Thyroid resistance

With thyroid resistance, your thyroid is working normally, but the hormones it's producing aren't getting where they're needed and you end up with hypothyroid symptoms. This pattern is usually caused by chronic high stress and high homocysteine. Unfortunately there is no test for thyroid resistance, and your standard labs will all come back "normal."

Hypothyroidism caused by pituitary dysfunction

High levels of cortisol, which can be caused by infection, blood sugar imbalances, stress, pregnancy, hypoglycemia, or insulin resistance, can fatigue the pituitary gland until it stops sending out the signal for your thyroid to release enough thyroid hormone. In this case, there might be nothing wrong with the thyroid itself, but rather with the pituitary gland.

If you have hypothyroid symptoms, your TSH falls below the functional range, but within the standard range, and T4 is low in the functional range, this may be your culprit.

Hypothyroidism caused by elevated TBG

Thyroid binding globulin (TBG) transports inactive thyroid hormone through the blood. If your TBG levels are too high, there won't be enough free thyroid hormone for your body to use.

High TBG levels are often caused by high estrogen levels, usually from birth control or estrogen replacement drugs. You have to get rid of the excess estrogen to clear this problem.

On your tests, TSH and T4 will be normal, but T3 will be low, and T3 uptake and TBG will be high.

Hypothyroidism caused by decreased TBG

The opposite of the previous pattern, too little TBG means that there's too much free thyroid hormone in your body—and your cells begin to develop resistance to it. So you will have hypothyroid symptoms.

You might guess that this is caused by too much testosterone in your system, and is often associated with PCOS and insulin resistance. Getting your blood sugars under control is key to healing this pattern

Your tests will show normal TSH and T4, but high T3. T3 uptake and TBG will be low.

Important takeaway: The patterns listed above don't show up on standard blood tests, and if one of those patterns is causing your thyroid imbalance, conventional thyroid hormone replacement will not be supportive to healing. That is the challenge with the way our current medical system addresses thyroid disease. It often skips the step of discovering the root cause of the imbalance and treats all thyroid healing the same usually through thyroid hormone replacement. When this method doesn't work for you, the doctor is left with the option of changing your medication or upping the dosage. If your thyroid disorder is caused by one of these patterns, neither treatment will be effective. You must treat the cause of the disorder in order to reverse the disease and eliminate symptoms and knowing the cause of the imbalance will set you on a path for success.

Rethinking Normal Ranges

So you had a test and you're "in the normal range." I'm sad to say, welcome to the club. Twelve doctors and two hospitals tested my thyroid and my levels were always in the "normal" ranges.

Fortunately, I finally received a comprehensive thyroid panel from a functional physician, which tested numerous factors that I'd never even heard about before. That is how I was finally diagnosed with Hashimoto's Thyroiditis.

I hadn't known that, while there are "normal lab values" for blood tests, there are also "FUNCTIONAL" or "OPTIMAL" values which actually tell you far more about your what's going on with your body (especially the thyroid). My TSH, T3, T4 and other basic thyroid levels have ALWAYS been in the "normal" range. However, when I was sick, they were not in the OPTIMAL ranges.

At **www.thyroidlovingcare.com/optimalranges**, you can download a list of functional/optimal ranges for thyroid markers and compare them to your latest blood test results.

From knowledge to healing.

It's no surprise that the butterfly is the symbol of the thyroid. In the literal sense, the thyroid itself is shaped like a butterfly...but in a deeper sense, the butterfly represents transformation. And transformation is exactly what you need for healing to occur.

You can find in literature on the ancient medical traditions of India (Ayurveda) and China (Traditional Chinese Medicine) that thyroid disease is believed to manifest when energy is blocked. From an emotional and energetic perspective, thyroid dysfunction is a disorder of the 5th chakra, or your body's center of communication. The 5th chakra gets blocked when we don't speak our truths and we don't speak up for ourselves. Due to this lack of open expression, it is believed that energy from this blockage will manifest itself as a thyroid disorder.

When you don't communicate your feelings, when you squash what's inside, your body reacts in ways to make you notice and put you back in balance. When you have Hashimoto's/ autoimmune thyroiditis, your body is literally attacking itself. It is attacking your thyroid, the seat of communication.

It makes sense, then (in a bigger, spiritual picture kind of way) that finding and using your voice, both literally and figuratively, can provide relief to your embattled thyroid. But it takes a transformation. You have to shed beliefs that don't serve you. You have to put your own needs in front of others sometimes. Due to this lack of open expression, it is believed that energy from this blockage will manifest itself as a thyroid disorder.

For many of us, this means a major shift in our mindset.

Almost all of the clients I see for thyroid and autoimmune disease have very similar characteristics. (I am including myself in this group!) Do any of these sound like you?

- We are type-A people who put pressure on ourselves to do it all.

- We are nurturers who take care of everyone else; often putting our own needs on the back burner.

- Most of us are self-admitted control freaks.

- Although type-A, we tend to really be shy, timid, or insecure. We worry about what others think of us.

- We tend to avoid conflict at all costs. We don't feel safe or comfortable in arguments and feel easily overpowered by others.

- When we try to confront others, we are either so choked up or blocked that we often feel isolated from others, even family.

- We often feel that there are things we cannot share about ourselves, such as our beliefs or life choices, and we have to hide who we really are because we want the love and approval of others.

- We may have experienced abuse or felt embarrassed by family members and felt we had to keep things hidden from others.

- We tend to be chatty Cathy's and drain our energetic reserves when in contact with others.

- We often crave attention and need to feel listened to, heard, appreciated, and understood.

- Because we have challenges in expressing ourselves directly, we tend to feel angry or resentful towards others because we cannot confront them and we feel like we don't have a voice.

From an emotional and energetic perspective, thyroid dysfunction is a communication disorder.

For me, getting back to singing as a hobby was a game changer. But you have to discover your own ways to find and use your voice.

There are many ways to start this transformation but first, you need to understand where you are starting from. We are all experiencing thyroid disease in a unique way. While most of us share the same symptoms, our bodies are reacting to these hormonal fluctuations and stress in different ways. For some of us, the illness manifests in adrenal burnout and thick fatigue, for others, it affects our guts and for others, it's anxiety and depression that crushes us daily.

We are all starting from a different place when healing thyroid disease. What stage of healing are you in?

After years of research and my own personal trial-and-error, I've discovered that there are really three phases of healing when it comes to thyroid diseases. Just like a caterpillar goes into the cocoon and emerges a brilliant butterfly, so do you as you move along your healing journey. So, I designed a free survey and report that you can take to understand fully where you're starting and what you can do to optimize healing.

What is transformation?

The butterfly develops through a process called **metamorphosis**. This is a Greek word that means **transformation.** For our purposes, healing is divided into three transformative phases: Caterpillar, Cocoon and Butterfly.

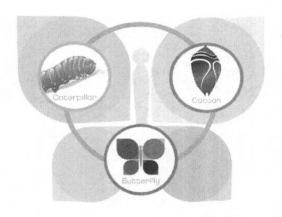

Phase 1: Caterpillar (The Nourishment Phase)

The job of the caterpillar is to eat and eat and eat....and that's your job too! The caterpillar is busy eating so it can nourish itself to prepare for the great transformation. But for us, when it comes to healing, it's not only eating that provides nourishment, it's also about nourishing our bodies and our minds. We need to do all three to begin repairing the body and to come back into balance. When you support your body by nourishing it so there is a foundation to heal, symptoms are relieved quickly and the disease can start to reverse itself.

Average time in the caterpillar phase: *6 weeks to 3 months.*

Of course, this all depends on your level of commitment and your desire to get well. When you make nourishing choices consistently, you'll find you can start eliminating symptoms quickly. If you're not consistent, you'll find it can take longer.

Discover if you're in the caterpillar phase and what you can do to support yourself today!

Phase 2: Cocoon (The Repair Phase)

After you've started nourishing your mind, body and spirit, you will start to notice some major changes in how you feel! Allergies will begin to subside, inflammation will decrease, symptoms will begin to disappear.

Now your body is ready to begin the repair process – and you head into the cocoon. The cocoon provides your body the protection it needs to heal. It may look like nothing is going on while you're in the cocoon phase but big changes are happening inside. You're about to get a boost in your energy, your hair may start coming in thicker, the mental fog clears and you get glimpses of feeling like yourself again.

At this point, you've done the work to eliminate symptoms and now it the body's time to repair what's at the root of the disease for you. For most people with Hashimoto's, you will be modulating the immune response, bringing adrenals into balance and repairing the gut. While you still have to be diligent in this phase, you will be able to add more foods back into your diet and can let up on your self-care schedule a bit (although you probably won't want to!).

Average time in the cocoon phase: *8 weeks to 6 months.*

Of course, this all depends on your level of commitment and the level of damage in your gut or adrenals. Stick to consistently making the nourishing choices and your body can repair itself quickly. Reverting to bad habits and not being consistent will make healing a slower process. Take care of you!

Discover if you're in the cocoon phase and what you can do to support yourself today!

Phase 3: Butterfly (The Freedom Phase)

Wow! This feels great, let me tell you! The Butterfly phase is where you can fly freely. You've emerged from the cocooned transformed!

You've made the nourishing choices and your body has repaired itself and come back into balance. You've addressed the root cause of your thyroid condition. Your energy is back, mind is clear, libido has returned. You feel "normal" again!

Blue skies ahead and you're flying through them.

In this phase, you can add most things back into your diet. This doesn't mean that you go back to your old ways and that you're free to abuse your body or your mind again. Do that and you'll find yourself right back in the same place. Be kind and gentle with yourself...as if you were holding a butterfly in your hand.

This is the time to stay diligent with your Radical TLC. Keep loving yourself. Keep up your self-care. Eat well so you can continue feeling great. You won't need reminding. You'll feel so great you'll want to keep it going...and, you'll be so in touch with your body's cues that you'll know when you're veering off course rather quickly.

In this phase, you've used all the tools at your disposal and you know which ones to pull out of your toolkit to bring you back to balance quickly. It's all about maintenance now, baby! You're free! **Take action <u>today</u>.**

Give Yourself Some TLC:

Ready to discover what phase of healing you're in?

I. Take the first step in your personal transformation from disease to dynamite by going to **www.freethyroidquiz.com** and get your FREE Thyroid Healing Type Quiz then write about your results.

II. Download the FREE digital journal (if you haven't already) at **www.yourbestthyroidlife.com/journal** and answer these questions.

A. Where are you in your healing phase?

B. What does it feel like to be a caterpillar?

C. What would it mean to cocoon for your health? To soar like a butterfly?

D. What will your life look like as you move through the next stages?

Healing with a feminine touch.

I'd love to take just a moment here to talk about how our western perspective treats illness in a very masculine way...we're supposed to "get over it," push through the pain or suffering, suffocate a symptom without ever processing what needs to be healed at the root. People with thyroid conditions often gain weight quickly and our society tells them to go on extreme diets and to push it at the gym or do cardio 'til they drop. This forceful way of approaching health care can keep us from healing.

When I first began my healing journey, I definitely felt at war with this disease and in a battle with my body. My approach at the time was to tackle the illness and to control everything. I tested and retested my blood. I tried to do everything "perfectly" and I lived and died by my blood test results. All the stress of trying to attack this disease was actually creating more imbalance and inflammation in the body and I couldn't shake my symptoms.

One day, I went to a doctor who also did energy work and I complained that I was "doing everything right" and that I was really angry at myself, my body and the universe because I wasn't getting any better. His advice to me? "Surrender. Stop trying to hold so tightly to the outcome of healing, to every blood test result, to every symptom. Surrender to the process of healing. It's a journey... and opening up to the understanding that your mind doesn't need to control everything because your body already knows how to heal itself is all you need to do."

Surrender.....hmmm. Not the easiest thing for a Type A-oholic to do but I realized that was the one thing I hadn't tried. Surrender.

So, I did that. And finally started seeing some lasting changes in my health.

Now I propose instead, that everyone (men and women!) approach their personal healthcare from the place of the feminine — nourishment, listening, and loving. When we tune into the body's cues and listen to what it has to say, when we support its repair and rebalancing through the nourishment it desires, and when we turn the love we readily give to others back unto ourselves, that's when true healing can begin.

Real Life TLC Success:
Helene, Age 40, Mother of 4, Professional

Helene became a client of mine after taking Thyroid Loving Care's free 15-day First Steps e-course to reverse thyroid, autoimmune and inflammatory conditions. She was dealing with all the emotional ups and downs of an over 15 year battle with Hashimoto's.

Helene worked with me as a private client participating in my one-day transformation intensive. During our day together, we covered healing, emotions, fitness and created custom meal and action plans for her.

Helene, busy balancing several children, a job and a husband who traveled for work often, was suffering with many symptoms including high antibody counts, insomnia, weight gain, adrenal fatigue, MTHFR, and serious digestive distress.

Helene was well researched and having battled with a thyroid condition for so long, she studied the topic so she knew and understood many of the techniques to reverse the disease...however, she hadn't gotten better throughout the years.

We utilized several different healing modalities and focused on balancing her medications and supplements to get her on the path toward healing. We also broke down all the obstacles she was facing in providing herself with the proper self-care and diet. What Helene needed most was a compassionate practitioner who would listen and customize care to her needs. Once she had hope again and had an accountability partner standing with her every step of the way, Helene began feeling better and her health improved.

CHAPTER 6

TLC in the Kitchen

HELLO, I'M JEN AND I'VE BEEN obsessed with food all my life. (*Hi Jen…*)

Are you like me? Do you eat, sleep and dream food too?

My love affair with food began where so many others have as well—around the kitchen table. I lucked out by having grandmothers who could really cook. My Nana's Italian sausages—a little spicy from the seasonings and sweet from rich tomato sauce—and my grandma Ida's comforting and nourishing chicken stew were both meals that could get me running to the table.

After graduating Valedictorian of my culinary school class (see: nerd + love of food), I started my own catering company and lived, cooked and worked in Italy for a year. Those were the good times.

After my accident, my body started to break down and I became allergic to all the foods I had loved and eaten before. I didn't know what I could eat to feel better and I truly didn't like any of the options. Food became a chore, the memory of enjoying it disappeared and everything felt like a giant "NO" sign.

I felt robbed—of my career, my mobility, my joy in food and my life.

Through a long year of diving deep into these emotions and a lot of trial and error in the kitchen, I finally figured out what worked best for my body… And then I figured out how to tweak my favorite dishes to fit my needs. All this tinkering brought back my passion for cooking, my zest for life and my desire to share my new knowledge of how to reverse thyroid, autoimmune and inflammatory disease through food.

This is the most literal part of the caterpillar phase of healing: NOURISHING your body with the right foods.

I went from eating and ENJOYING a biscuit and gravy Midwestern diet of bread, cheese, more bread and added sugar to eating and ENJOYING a diet rich in fresh, organic fruits and veggies, meats from animals that get to live outside, feeding on green pasture, fish that are wild caught and high quality fats.

Does that scare you? Don't worry; it's a pretty common reaction. It's hard to imagine giving up something that's been such a huge part of your life, that ties you to people in your family and your community, that maybe even feels like it defines part of you.

Maybe you're already thinking that you couldn't possibly make that big of a change in your diet. Maybe you're remembering times in your past when you tried to go on a diet and didn't get the results you wanted. (And maybe — MAYBE — ended up face down in a box of powdered sugar doughnuts, not that I would know anything about that!)

But this way of eating and living is not about deprivation, it's about reparation. It's not about willpower, but the power of loving yourself back to health, repairing the years of damage from eating the SAD (Standard American Diet). Repairing the gut lining so you can metabolize food properly and absorb important nutrients and minerals. Repairing your body so you can support your thyroid and manage your weight.

And the real bonus? You get all of this with quick, delicious meals that are simple to make and will never leave you hungry.... I never have to count calories or watch my portion size. I eat as much of this goodness as I want and feel better every day.

My Leaky Gut

Sounds gross, doesn't it? But "leaky gut" is a phrase that came up a lot when I was first learning about my Hashimoto's disease and how to heal.

The popular quote by Hippocrates, **"Let food be thy medicine and medicine be thy food,"** could not ring more true. In order for our bodies to heal, we must provide them with the nourishment they need through whole, unprocessed foods. But, what happens to healing when your body isn't absorbing the nourishing foods properly?

Hippocrates also said, **"All disease begins in the gut,"** and that's where we'll start this story. If your body isn't functioning properly, disease will be able to creep in and take hold. Poor gut health is intricately connected to low thyroid function and additionally can trigger Hashimoto's disease.

When your thyroid isn't working properly, it causes inflammation and causes your immune system to go into overdrive, which in turns causes a leaky gut. The leaky gut then causes more inflammation and immune dysregulation which further harms the thyroid. Press repeat. The cycle of destruction is endless if it is not addressed.

An inflamed and leaky gut contributes to just about every disease out there. Without healing the gut, you cannot truly heal the thyroid or begin to address the many (MANY) symptoms that can go along with it.

The gut is host to 70% of your immune tissue in your body. These tissues store immune cells that carry out attacks and produce antibodies if there is a foreign invader or potential threats. That's a really good function if you have a bacteria or virus coming in for attack. However, when these protective functions are compromised, the intestinal barrier becomes permeable (leaky) meaning stuff escapes through it into the bloodstream.

Since food proteins (like casein, gluten, et al) don't belong outside of the gut, the body initiates an immune response and attacks them. (This is what creates an "allergic" response or food sensitivity.) The problem comes in when the body turns the attack on itself in response to the protein (think gluten) and, as in the case of Hashimoto's, inadvertently attacks the thyroid gland. Studies have shown that these attacks are linked to the development of all types of autoimmune disease.

Tight junctions keep the barrier of the stomach and small intestine impermeable; meaning that proteins can't pass through. That's what we want. Thyroid hormones strongly influence the tight junctions in the gut. However, when thyroid health is compromised, the gut can become inflamed leading to further permeability just continuing the cycle.

Inflammation in the gut also increases cortisol levels, and too much cortisol in the system presents a cascading set of challenges including weight gain and further thyroid degeneration.

Another component to healing a leaky gut is having the right gut-bacteria balance. Bacteria in the gut actually assist in converting 20% of inactive T4 into the active form of T3. This is what we use to balance our body's metabolic functions. This is what we need to have good energy, feel right in our bodies and to keep our weight stable.

Major Takeaway: There are five major reasons that you need to love your gut back to health in order to heal your thyroid:

1. There needs to be a balance of beneficial bacteria in the gut to make your thyroid hormone levels work right.

2. We need to keep stress and inflammation low in order to heal our bodies.

3. We need to reverse the autoimmune response.

4. Low stomach acid increases intestinal permeability which is linked with autoimmune thyroid disease. It is also associated with GERD, inflammation and infection.

5. Constipation can impair hormone clearance and cause elevations in estrogen causing problems with the thyroid. It also increases inflammation, infections and doesn't allow for proper absorption in the gut.

As you can see, you can't have a healthy gut without a healthy thyroid, and you can't have a healthy thyroid without a healthy gut. To boost thyroid function and heal your gut, you have to address both simultaneously.

Healing a leaky gut isn't something that can happen overnight. (That's the bad news.) The good news is that it CAN be healed. But it requires some change.

It's a "live-it" not a diet.

The flat truth is, I didn't *want* to change my lifestyle because of my disease. It's a hard pill to swallow. At the very beginning, I tried to convince myself that I could live with "less" of the things I was supposed to give up: cut back on sugar, eat less bread, etc. But, not surprisingly, I wasn't getting the kind of results I wanted.

A lot of the research out there supports going on a very extreme/limited diet in order to heal. However, I've found that these wonderfully healing diets can not only be intimidating and overwhelming, but they are hard to do when you're first beginning your healing journey.

So, instead of diving into the GAPS protocol or the Autoimmune Paleo protocol, I have found with myself and my clients that we see better results when we make small dietary shifts first and as we add more shifts, we move slowly closer to the "ideal" healing diet.

Here's the truth: it's hard to make big changes when you feel like crap! But when you can make a small change, you feel a small bit better. As we start to feel better and gain more energy, it's easier to embark on these truly healing protocols—but one step at a time!

The approach I embraced is a lifestyle plan, not a diet. We all know diets don't work—because the very idea of "going on a diet" implies that you will go off it sooner or later. Unlike with a "diet," I've found that I don't *want* to cheat or go off plan, because I feel so much better eating the way I do on the plan.

When you commit to following a meal plan that is supportive for Hashimoto's disease, you can see results in terms of less weight and bloat within a matter of days! You'll start to see disease reversal in a matter of weeks or months as your symptoms disappear.

And remember, reversing disease is a lifestyle itself — you've got to not only put thought into what you eat but you have to support yourself with fitness and stress relief (which we'll talk about later).

I believe in understanding what foods our bodies need to heal, stocking our fridge with those foods and then forgetting about the "rules." Once you get your kitchen and your routines set up to support your healing, you can pretty much forget about your diet! It will take care of itself.

There are three big steps I took to heal my body at first, and they were cutting out sugar, ditching gluten, and modeling my meals on a Paleo meal plan.

Real Life TLC Success:
Nathalie, Age 65, Artist & Designer

Nathalie had been suffering with Hashimoto's, an autoimmune thyroid condition, for over 40 years! She became a client of mine upon a recommendation of a family friend. Her main issue was diet. She was fit but wasn't feeding herself enough and struggled with insomnia, brain fog and fatigue. Because she and her husband dined out often, she felt she didn't have enough control over her food and didn't understand what you could eat while dining out that would be nourishing.

We also worked on Nathalie"s schedule as she was a classic Type-A who often wouldn't take a break for lunch or for a moment to just breathe. So we focused on lifestyle design, time management, self-care and devised strategies for meals at work and when dining out. After just a few sessions together, Nathalie made huge improvements and reversed her symptoms. She was able to sleep well again, her brain fog lifted and her mood improved.

Saying Sayonara To Sugar

When we're making big changes, it helps to get a little instant (or almost instant) success to make us feel good and keep us going. Limiting sugar is one of the fastest ways to see results when you're trying to heal your Hashimoto's.

Ditching the sugar reduces inflammation, helps your body balance blood sugar levels, keeps insulin and leptin resistance at bay, decreases digestive troubles, reduces brain fog, and helps you metabolize better so you can lose weight and improve your mood!

Doesn't that sound amazing??

But I'm not going to sugar-coat this: It's not exactly easy as pie.

A few years ago, I attended a health Mega Conference in Long Beach where I was absolutely shocked to learn from one of the speakers that sugar is actually 4 times as addictive as cocaine. What? Four times more addictive than what!?! I couldn't believe it but the proof literally is in the pudding. With Diabetes escalating every day and waistlines ever expanding, it is not only clear in research experiments but also to the naked eye, that we have an addiction to sugar in the U.S.

Sugar is pervasive in our American diet. All kinds of foods that you would not associate with sugar have been processed with this other "white powder." Did you know that taco seasoning and tomato sauce contain added sugars?

When I finally took the plunge and quit sugar, my health improved immediately. Once you quit, you don't crave sweets as much and when you do take a bite of dessert, a bite is all you actually need to feel satisfied.

However, when I decided to quit sugar, Valentine's Day was just a few weeks ago. My husband wanted to be sweet and brought home a small tub of coconut macaroons for me. It's really the only treat I could eat without having a reaction due to all of my food sensitivities. It started out as one bite of one macaroon. At first I thought they were too sweet. I went back for another bite then another macaroon and then another.

During the next few days, I was exhausted. I started adding caffeine and more sugar to my diet. Within the week, my face had broken out with acne, I was severely dehydrated and I had a systemic Candida infection. All of this from one bite of an ultra sugary macaroon.

Can you say addictive? That's right – four times as addictive as cocaine! It happened to me and I had withdrawal symptoms for two days after I decided to stop the sugar roller-coaster madness. I've now been free of my sugar addiction for years. My acne and Candida have subsided, I'm able to sleep better and I'm full of energy. Plus, I lost a few pounds off of the tummy tire I had acquired during my sugar binge. I learned my lesson!

I'm not perfect. I'm a Health Coach who fell prey to the siren call of sugar but at least I had the tools to reign it back in quickly. It's amazing the power sugar can have over your mind — and your body.

Unfortunately, on a general level, sugar inhibits all healing. Sugar creates inflammation, turns off your body's appetite-control function, leads to weight gain and belly fat, feeds candida and has a host of additional toxic effects. All of that sounds terrible enough but it gets worse.

What does this mean for your thyroid?

Many people with thyroid dysfunction seem to be especially sensitive to refined sugars or even consuming too many natural sugars. When you constantly consume sugar, you literally burn out your adrenal and thyroid glands. There is a risk of damaging or even destroying the thyroid. If you don't reduce or eliminate sugar in the diet, there is a risk for permanent damage and that's no good!

Sugar can also affect your mood and energy levels.

Are you always hungry? Do you get bouts of dizziness, nervousness, a racing heartbeat, shakiness or sweating? Do you feel like you could turn into the Incredible Hulk if you miss a meal?

If any of these resonate with you, you could have an issue with your blood sugar. Keeping your blood sugar regulated is crucial to healthy thyroid function and to keep your blood sugar in a normal range your thyroid needs to be functioning properly. Whether your blood sugar is too low or too high, it can create issues for the thyroid. When your blood sugar isn't regulated it will take its toll on your body in the form of:

- high blood pressure

- inflammation

- abdominal obesity

- high cholesterol and triglycerides

- insulin resistance

- tendency to form blood clots

Blood sugar surges, which can cause insulin resistance, increase the destruction of the thyroid in people with Hashimoto's disease. The more destruction that occurs in the gland, the more thyroid hormone production falls.

When your blood sugar is chronically low, cortisol (the stress hormone) is repeatedly released, which suppresses pituitary function. If your pituitary gland isn't functioning properly, the thyroid won't function properly either.

Blood sugar regulation is crucial to healing. If you don't stabilize your blood sugar, your thyroid will not be able to heal.

How to release the weight

One of the quickest ways to get control of your weight and balance your body's blood sugar/insulin processes again is by cutting sugar out of your diet. Even if you currently only eat "natural" sugars from fruit, honey, agave nectar, you could still be ingesting an enormous amount per day.

You don't have to cut sugar out of your diet forever; fruits definitely have some health benefits, as does raw honey. But by eliminating sugar from your diet for a short period of time, when you're first starting to heal, you give your body the chance to learn to regulate your blood sugar levels, to heal, to get a better sense of when you're actually hungry, and increase your immune system's ability to fight off illness and ward off Candida infections.

Goodbye Gluten

Remember how I said I'm from the Midwest? And how I *love* all things Italian (like the three Ps: pasta, pizza and pastry)?

Imagine my reaction when I found out I was going to have to give up my beloved bread to heal.

A bit deflated, as you can believe! Before I started living gluten-free, I wasn't sure how I would ever succeed. But I *did* succeed. (And honey, if I can do it, so can you!)

Gluten molecules resemble thyroid tissue. What does this mean to you? It means that if you have intestinal permeability (leaky gut) or a sensitivity to gluten, your body will mistakenly attack your thyroid believing it is attacking the gluten molecules.

What happens with autoimmune disease is that the body is having an overactive immune response against substances and tissues normally present in the body. In addition, the thyroid gland is connected to so many of the body's systems including gastrointestinal function, stomach acid production, adrenal hormone metabolism, changes in brain chemistry and liver detoxification. So, when a gluten molecule escapes through the walls of the digestive tract and the body starts attacking the gluten, it inadvertently begins to attack the thyroid as well, continuing its destruction.

That's pretty serious stuff. Some doctors and thyroid researchers insist that if you want to stop the destruction of the thyroid, you must stop eating gluten.

You may have heard all of this before, but now is the time to start acting on it. If you truly want to heal your thyroid condition, you've got to love your body enough to put your hands up and drop the croissant.

I learned loads of tips and tricks and have a host of new recipe resources to boot. I began feeling so much better after parting ways with gluten that I don't even feel like I need it anymore. Sure, a piece of fresh-baked bread smells delightful, but my body doesn't actually crave it anymore.

"How can I give up my pasta or pizza? What will I eat instead?" you wonder. "Will I ever be full?"

I promise you will, and there are loads of delicious, naturally gluten-free foods out there. Giving up gluten seems unappealing and daunting, I know. But you can shift your thinking from giving something up to *gaining* something: your health.

This is not an act of self-deprivation, my friend; <u>it is an act of self-love</u>.

Hello Paleo

All caveman jokes aside, it turns out that a meal plan based on the popular Paleo diet is actually pretty close to perfect for healing Hashimoto's. It cuts out the foods that are inflaming the gut and exacerbating your thyroid condition, and encourages foods that promote healing.

I know, I know. Are you worried about being one of "those" people? The ones who have to make ridiculously complicated orders at restaurants and then dine with an air of superiority and smugness?

It doesn't have to be that way. The Paleo approach I take can be described by that famous Michael Pollan quote: "Eat food. Not too much. Mostly plants."

Sound doable? It is! Imagine a gorgeous, fresh salad topped with grilled chicken and avocado in a silky homemade vinaigrette. Or braised beef spare ribs with buttery soft roasted veggies. Or a huge platter of lamb kabobs, fresh cucumber and tomato salad, and rich olives…. (Now I'm getting hungry!)

Eating the way the Paleo diet suggests also comes with a wide range of benefits *in addition* to the benefits to your thyroid, including:

- Increased and more stable energy levels

- Improved sleep

- Clearer skin and healthier looking hair

- Mental clarity

- Improved mood and attitude

- Improvements in those suffering depression or anxieties

- Less or no bloating, decreased gas

- Sustained weight loss

- Muscle growth; increased fitness

- Lowered risk of heart disease, diabetes and cancer

- Higher immune function and a general feeling of well being

- Improved glucose tolerance; decreased insulin secretion and increased insulin sensitivity

- Improved lipid profiles

- Healthier gut flora

- Better absorption of nutrients from food

- Reduced allergies

- Paleo diet is anti-inflammatory, most people experience reduction of pain associated with inflammation

- Improvements in those with respiratory problems such as asthma

Of course, while the healing meal plan I suggest is inspired by Paleo, I believe we should always take the best and leave the rest. I don't think strict adherence to a Paleo diet is the right fit for everyone. Plus, there are almost as many variations of the Paleo or primal diet as there are books and experts out there!

Here's what I do: I believe in veggie heavy Paleo eating. Your meals should consist of loads of vegetables with a side of meat. Yes, a side of meat and not the other way around. I found that when the diet gets too meat heavy, my body and my system get a little sluggish and stinky (I won't go into all of the dirty details). The point is that, although I felt better overall, I didn't feel great when I was eating too much meat.

Now, don't get me wrong, I am a lover of meat, especially my dear friend, bacon. But I noticed a huge difference when I turned the Paleo diet upside down and made my plates consist of 75–80% organic veggies, 10–15% pastured, grass-fed or wild-caught meat, and 10% fats from avocados, olives, coconut oil, butter from pastured cows and from properly processed nuts and seeds.

You may need to tweak those percentages a bit for your own body but going veggie heavy is, in my opinion, the way to approach the Paleo plan. Believe in the intuition of YOUR body to let you know what feels best to it. Basically, all you need to do is eat real, whole food including organic fruits and veggies, healthy fats, pastured or wild-caught meats and nothing processed or packaged. It's not hard and it's so delicious and filling.

Real Life TLC Success:
Dawn, 40, Mother & Business Owner

Dawn came in with adrenal fatigue, severe hair loss, leaky gut, fatigue, a thyroid imbalance and a Vitamin D and iron deficiency. We focused on diet, exercise and relaxation techniques tailored to fit into Dawn's busy lifestyle as a mom and business owner.

When Dawn initially began working with me, she was following a very low protein meal plan. My gut told me that Dawn really needed to incorporate red meat into her diet. This was something that she wasn't inclined to do - red meat actually turned her stomach. So, we worked together to create a meal plan that would slowly re-introduce red meat to her diet in appetizing ways. Within a couple of weeks, her energy was WAY up and she was enjoying the new diet. Over time, we were able to reverse the hair loss and talked about ways to work self-care into an overwhelming schedule. Dawn's blood levels have now improved and her life was transformed by making the necessary dietary and lifestyle changes that supported her healing.

A day on my "diet"

So, just in case you're still wondering, here's what a day on my healing "diet" looks like:

- **Breakfast:** I keep it really simple in my house and

personally eat a filling bowl of chicken soup or pho (a popular Vietnamese soup) and two Brazil nuts every morning. I'll eat eggs or a GF version of a traditional breakfast on the weekends on occasion. The pho just feels so good in my belly and it's rich in minerals and anti-inflammatory spices.

- **Lunch:** For lunches and dinners an ideal meal would consist of two cooked veggies, a salad with some good-fat toppings like avocado, and a high-quality protein. The easiest way to get that? Make enough dinner so you have leftovers for lunch! I'm always eating leftovers or a giant salad for lunch.

- **Snack:** If I feel hungry between meals, I usually grab a piece of fresh fruit and some olives, nuts and veggie sticks.

- **Dinner:** My most creative meal of the day! I don't let my health hold me back. I love to cook up dinners like chicken piccata, BBQ short ribs, or butter chicken for dinner—and make sure there's enough to enjoy tomorrow.

I always encourage my clients not to focus on what they *can't* have, but on all the amazing things they *can* have. I know you can take on this lifestyle change and heal your body, because I've seen so many of my friends and clients do it for themselves.

And if this Italy-loving, Midwestern chef can do it—so can you!

The Super Simple TLC Thyroid & Autoimmune Diet Strategy

So, now that we know more about the foods that are halting your healing, creating a menu plan that's simple and healthy for you and your family is not as hard as you think. With a couple of tried and true tricks and a systematic approach, you can have healthy meals for you and your family in a snap!

Start by stocking your pantry first, as this is the foundation to eating healthy. If you don't have the right foods in ready supply, it's too simple to grab those pesky, problematic go-to foods when cravings rear their ugly heads or hunger arrives. Having a pantry and refrigerator stocked with easy healthy food for you and your family is the way to go.

Next, create a master list of favorite foods and favorite recipes. Write down foods you love that also just happen to be healthy. It can be divided into categories—starchy vegetables, non-starchy vegetables, fruit, meats, nuts, canned and other. Under each category list of your favorite foods that you can pull from when creating your weekly menu.

From the favorites list, create a weekly menu plan including breakfasts, lunches, and dinners. For breakfasts, choose 1-3 favorites and rotate them throughout the week. For dinners, choose a starchy vegetable, a non-starchy vegetable, salad ingredients, and a meat and fat to comprise the dinner meal. Choose a fruit off the favorites list for dessert and save your leftovers for lunch.

Creating a menu plan helps you save money, reduce food waste and creates a system so you only have to shop once a week. With the favorites list already created, it makes menu planning a snap! Want buy-in from your kids? Let them in on the menu planning by giving them one or two days a week where they get to plan the meal.

Now, that you have your menu plan, preparing your grocery list will be a piece of cake (just don't add cake to your grocery list!). Just go through each meal and each day of your menu plan and write out the ingredients you need to create the meal. Having a list at the grocery store will keep you honest, on track, and will save you time while shopping. You'll end up buying healthier ingredients and keep those harmful foods out of your cart.

And be sure to only shop when you're full! Going on an empty stomach is a recipe for disaster. You might also enlist friends or family members to take care of the kids so you can shop alone.

Having a healthy and simple menu plan for you and your family can make mealtime a breeze. It not only keeps your budget in check, it reduces food waste and time spent at the grocery store. And, don't forget the most important part—menu planning can help your waistline and general wellness so you can make good choices to support your health, energy and vitality.

Give Yourself Some TLC:

How does your food *really* make you feel? Most people don't have a clue. Try keeping a food journal for a couple of days — ideally a week. Start with what you ate and when, and then include how you feel at different times of the day.

When you go back and read through your entries, you might discover trends. Does your doughnut wear off and leave you starving by 10am? Is your 3pm slump preceded by a carb-heavy lunch? Do you crave sweets when you get home from work, or when the kids are going crazy?

Before you make any changes to your diet, I think it's important for you to see for yourself how your diet is changing you.

Real Life TLC Success:
Peggy, Age 47, Stay-at-home Mom

Peggy worked with me through my online group coaching program, The Thyroid Fix in 6. She joined the program so she could manage weight and relieve symptoms. Peggy was dealing with a tough case of adrenal stress and had tried almost everything out there. Within the first 4 weeks of the program, Peggy lost 22 lbs. Through our live group coaching calls where we'd troubleshoot obstacles clients were facing, we worked directly on incorporating self-care into Peggy's schedule and on designing a better fitness program that would allow her to restore adrenal function while continuing to lose weight and get fit.

CHAPTER 7

Self-Care and Healing

THE HARDEST AND MOST rewarding thing I did for my health was making self-care a part of my routine.

Yup. You read that right. Giving up gluten, cutting out sugar, ditching soy, going Paleo — none of that was hard compared to climbing over the mental barrier I had erected against taking time for myself.

The first and most important step to healing is practicing self-love. It may sound hokey if you're used to taking care of everyone but yourself, but that, my dear friend, is likely how you got here. It's time for a change; remember that you can't take care of anyone until you take care of yourself.

It's vital to ensure that the body is getting enough sleep, detoxifying itself properly, and that healing functions are being supported in every way possible.

But this step is particularly hard for so many people — especially women. They're not used to putting themselves first.

Loving yourself means letting others in

It takes a village when it comes to healing, literally. And, you need people on your team. You've already got one member of your team—that's me! But your friends and family are your most important allies in healing. For people like us, asking for help can be hard, and it might require that you get vulnerable but it's important to do. You have to let people in, explain how this disease causes you suffering, talk about your plan to heal and ask them to be part of your healing team—to hold you accountable to your commitment to creating new habits that will help you heal and ask them not to tempt you or sabotage your efforts by undermining this goal. By letting people in, you will get more support than you can imagine and that boost will help you make it across the finish line even quicker—it's a victory for everyone!

If you're having trouble finding the words to let people into this world of thyroid or autoimmune dysfunction, please use the letter below to help your friends and family have a better understanding. They want to help, they just might not know how.

Dear _____,

As you may know, I have been dealing with [insert your diagnosis here]. It's a disorder that attacks my thyroid—but more than that, it attacks every aspect of my life. It is an invisible disease; most of the time, other people can't see my symptoms, but they're always there, and they're very real.

Every system in our bodies is influenced by our

thyroid, and so this disease can cause a whole range of symptoms. It can cause insomnia, or make me want to sleep all day. It can cause me to gain weight and be unable to lose it, no matter what I do. It can suck all the energy I have right out of me, and leave me dealing with intense pain or a deep ache all over. It can even make me feel anxious or depressed

And those are just *some* of the symptoms. The list goes on and on.

Because it affects every part of my body, it's very hard to diagnose and even harder to treat. I know that it's also hard for anyone who isn't me to understand what I'm going through. It may have seemed like I was complaining in the past, or making a mountain out of a molehill, but what I have is real, and it's not going away without a fight and some serious self-care.

The good news is that I have decided to take control. I'm making a lot of lifestyle changes that can help me heal, and I need your help—I hope you will be a part of my healing team. First of all, I just need your understanding and support. If you want to know more about my disease, I would be happy to tell you.

Second, if I ask you for some help, I need you to understand that it's because I'm doing everything in my power to heal myself, not because I'm lazy or malingering. If you can't help, that's OK! Just the understanding will be huge.

It means so much to me to have your support right now.

{SIGNED, YOU}

The caterpillar, cocoon and butterfly phases of healing aren't just about nourishing your body literally with the proper food, it's also about nourishing your mind and soul. One thing I truly believe Western medicine has gotten wrong is that we treat ailments all on their own — as though they are separate from the rest of the body. But the body is a whole, and we have to treat the whole in order to heal.

While I was writing this book, I reflected on what this journey has been about for me personally, and realized that this has really been about learning to fall in love with myself again. The common thread connecting myself and my clients are that we are people who nurture everyone else in our lives but we aren't great about nurturing ourselves. We're often Type-A people who need to control and do everything ourselves with little help from others... But, we're the first people called when someone needs love, support, friendship, and so on.

All that is great, except somewhere along the way, we've forgotten that we're worthy and deserving of the same love we show others. And when you are diagnosed with a thyroid disorder, it gets worse... Your body turns on you, you feel and/ or get fat, you don't like yourself, your mind, your body, the way you feel, your energy level, your inability to do what others do (to feel normal), etc.

Hashimoto's can take you on a journey to self-loathing

and that's where I bottomed out before I picked myself up and decided I was determined to heal. What I learned was that I had to love myself and my body again. That we couldn't be at war with each other. I had to love my thyroid, respect it and give it compassionate care in order to heal. I had to work with my body again (in partnership) and show it love through proper nourishment and self-care.

The self-care practices I discovered on my own journey and that I suggest to my clients help address some of these problems that so many of us encounter. They open us up to opportunities to feel appreciated, they liberate us to put ourselves first for a change, and help us discover our true voice. Some of these practices may sound like luxuries at first, because our society puts so little stock in preventive care. But I assure you: they are important and necessary to your healing.

The rate of women ignoring their own needs in favor of their families is epidemic. I know you've seen it (even if you aren't ready to admit your own culpability yet!): the mom who lets herself go, whose kids look like little fashion plates while she's wearing jeans from the 1990s, the martyr who has given up *everything* for her family (and probably lets you know about it at every opportunity).

But why do we do it?

Fitting in with traditional roles

The traditional roles of wife and mother that many of us

want to take on are all about caring for others. In fact, it's so ingrained into our psyches that many times women who don't have a significant other or children still end up playing a caregiver role somewhere in their lives.

Add to that the stresses of working outside the home for some women, and taking care of ourselves ends up feeling like just one more "job." This is especially true when you have Hashimoto's disease, and taking care of everyone else uses up every last bit of energy you have.

Competition

We all do it. We look around the carpool lane, the office, PTA night, and mentally slot the women we see into categories. *She's got it all together.*

Society and the media tell us that we need to have it "all together" and we judge ourselves if we feel overwhelmed. We see other women that seem to have it all together and we fear we don't measure up. It's easy to feel inadequate when we think everyone else is handling life better than we are! But what often ends up happening is that women "drop out" of the game as they see it, which makes it "ok" not to take care of themselves.

Fear

Sometimes we stop caring for ourselves because of a bigger,

deeper fear. It might be a fear of rejection or a fear of accepting how you really are. It could be a fear that, deep down, you aren't "enough." It could be fear of how others see you.

This fear tells women to let other people decide their self-worth.

If you saw yourself in any of these reasons, don't despair! You're not alone; in fact, you're sadly pretty normal in today's society. But that doesn't mean you have to stay in this place of self-deprivation.

Your internal compass that directs your life needs recalibrating; but just like butterflies can migrate hundreds of miles to find the perfect place to live their lives, you can also learn to follow your internal compass to self-care and happiness.

What does self-care look like?

At first, my self-care routine felt awkward and forced. Some days it was like pulling teeth to make myself sit down and write in my journal or meditate. Some weeks, the thought of finding time to go get a massage felt like *one more thing to do.*

As with anything worth doing, self-care takes practice. We've forgotten how to take care of ourselves and it's a skill that has to be relearned step by step.

What's important to remember is that these practices aren't just *woo-woo-out-there-feel-good-B.S.* The self-care practices I have used for myself and recommend to my clients are scientifically proven to help you heal.

Just like with making changes to your diet, I found that the best way for me to relearn self-care was to introduce strategies slowly, one at a time, until I built up a routine that worked with my life to support my health.

Give Yourself Some TLC:

Take 5 minutes to write in your journal:

1. How have you let your own self-care slip?

2. Are there things you used to do (yoga class, exercise, hobbies, hair appointments, spa days, etc.) that you stopped doing?

3. Why did you stop?

4. What stories are you telling yourself about why you "can't" take care of yourself?

Sleep

How many times have you found yourself staring up at the ceiling in the middle of the night, praying that you could just fall asleep? You're completely exhausted and your body needs to rest but nothing happens. And by nothing, I mean your thoughts race incessantly and you toss and turn as you try to will your body to sleep. Or, you sleep for 10 hours and still wake up completely exhausted. Does this sound like you?

There was a time when I hadn't slept in three years. I had a terrible time sleeping while I was pregnant, as my thyroid disease was undiagnosed, and then I didn't get the chance to sleep for the first two years of my son's life. Somehow, I kept getting up and making it through the day, but I was running on empty.

For our body to restore itself, we must rest fully each day. For some reason in our culture, we tend to pride ourselves on how much we're able to accomplish without having to sleep. When people have had a rough night, they sometimes engage in a competition as to who had the worst night sleep or who slept the least. It's as if it is a badge of honor or something to brag about. But, this is no contest to win!

Poor sleep is a typical symptom for people with Hashimoto's and often it is just accepted as something you have to live with as part of having the disease. The problem is that insomnia or restless sleep must be addressed so that your endocrine system can be supported in order to heal.

We can't be flippant about a sleep disorder. Too often, it's accepted, solely medicated or totally disregarded. Discovering the most effective way to get to sleep and sleep well is a must for loving yourself back to health. Here's why:

1. Sleep loss can cause weight gain.

2. Lack of sleep can make you feel depressed.

3. Sleep deprivation can lead to serious health problems like heart disease, heart attack, heart failure, irregular heartbeat, high blood pressure, stroke, diabetes.

4. Lack of sleep affects libido.

5. Sleepiness impairs judgments and makes you prone to/ causes accidents.

6. Sleep loss affects intellect and memory.

7. Lack of sleep ages your skin. (Yikes!)

Sound familiar? A lot of the symptoms of not getting enough sleep mirror the symptoms of thyroid and autoimmune disease, so you must make sure you're getting enough sleep to be sure that your symptoms aren't being caused or exacerbated by exhaustion.

What's most important to know?

- **You should maintain a regular sleep-wake schedule.** I did this by trying to go to bed 15 minutes earlier each night for 5 nights until I was able to fall asleep by 10pm.

I also set my alarm for 6am each day so I could exercise. After 3 days on the 10pm–6am schedule, I was hooked and it was easy to stick to.

- **Avoid caffeine, alcohol, nicotine, and other chemicals that interfere with sleep.** I can't stress this enough. I know you're tired now in the morning so you like your cup of coffee but giving it up could be the difference between sleepless nights and sound rest. I went from drinking coffee several times a day to doing a caffeine detox. I don't need or crave caffeine anymore. It's pretty amazing.

- **Make your bedroom a comfortable sleep environment.** Keep your bedroom uncluttered and cozy with the right bedding, blankets and a heater (if you need it).

- **Establish a calming pre–sleep routine.** For instance, read something spiritual, inspirational or meditative before bed. It's actually a great time to do a 10–15 minute meditation.

- **Go to sleep when you're tired** Don't stay up to watch the end of that TV show or keep reading to finish a chapter. Research shows that our body wakes itself up after 10pm. Once you're up later in the night, you'll get a second wind and may struggle with falling asleep altogether.

- **Keep lights low in the evening.** Bright household lights and light from computers and other electronic devices can disrupt messengers in your brain from eliciting the sleep response.

- **Don't nap close to bedtime.** Eating a light meal really helps with this one. When you eat a heavy, carb laden dinner, you produce chemicals which make you sleepy. Taking a nap after dinner is gonna make it hard to fall asleep when it's best for your body.

Six to eight hours of restful sleep each night is crucial for maximum rejuvenation. Interestingly, studies have shown that your body is able to rejuvenate better if you fall asleep in the hours before midnight. Meaning, if you are sleeping eight hours between 10pm—6am, you will feel more rested than if you slept eight hours between Midnight and 8 am. I can attest to that as I've tested it out myself. If I fall asleep by 10pm, I can jump out of bed at 6am and am actually energized enough to exercise. When I stay up late watching TV or reading and go to sleep at 11 or 11:30pm, I'll drag in the morning even if I'm sleeping the same amount of time.

I want you to try setting yourself a sleep schedule and sticking to it. If you feel resistance to this, ask yourself why. Make a list of the best excuses you can think of, and then ask yourself, "Is X more important than my health?" Be honest with yourself and remember that loving yourself enough to give yourself what you need is the key to healing.

Massage

How often do you get a massage?

Massage is so much more than just a luxury. It's true that it's something you have to invest in, but as with so many of the steps you're taking towards healing, it's an investment in your long-term health and wellbeing.

Medical studies have revealed that even a 10 or 20 minute massage (the kind you can get at the grocery store or the mall!) can have therapeutic benefits including: improving immune function, boosting circulation, reducing stress, reducing the time it takes to recover from injury, and alleviating pain. It can also reduce depression and anxiety and promote restful sleep patterns.

This is huge for Hashimoto's sufferers! Stress, depression, and sleeplessness are three of the toughest symptoms I see my community struggle with time and time again. If they are symptoms you experience, I urge you to take the free thyroid quiz to see where you fall on the spectrum.

Massage also promotes circulation and the elimination of toxins from your body, which are key to improving your thyroid health. The reason I had to change my diet in order to heal my thyroid was to stop introducing toxins into my body, but when you're struggling with thyroid disease, very often part of the problem is that those toxins have built up in your system over time, and you have to take steps to clear the old toxins out. Massage is one of the best (and most enjoyable!) ways to do that.

And, massage is making its way into "mainstream" medical treatment. Some insurance policies now cover massage, and some massage chains (like Massage Envy) are adept at filing claims with your insurance company for you.

Remember, this is about your long-term health; I believe it's worth taking a look at the budget to see where a professional massage might fit in the way you would fit in your prescription medications or doctor's visits. But, if the investment is a concern, you can look for a massage school in your area, which usually provide massage services at a discount. And, whether you're on a budget or just looking to include massage in your daily self-care routine, you can try these two self-massage techniques at home:

Self-Massage to Improve Sleep:

- Place the three fingers of each hand on your eyebrows. Close your eyes and take a few deep, cleansing breaths.

- Using your middle fingers, start at the bridge of your nose and move along the line of your brows, rubbing small slow circles, all the way to your temples.

- Repeat several times, each time moving your fingers up a little ways until you are following your hair line.

- Follow your hairline all the way around the the nape of your neck, making small circles. Repeat this several times.

- Using the same circular movements, move from the nape of your neck down the back of your neck, on either side of (but not on) your spine.

- Start in the center of your forehead and make these circular movements back, across your scalp, to the nape of your neck.

- Finally, using your entire hand, knead your scalp gently.

Self Foot Massage:

- It's best to start this right after a bath, but not totally necessary.

- Start in a comfortable sitting position with your right foot propped up on your left knee so that you can see the sole of your foot.

- Use a few drops of lotion or massage oil and wrap your hands around your foot. Using your thumbs, make strong circular motions from the heel of your foot all the way up to your toes.

- Use your thumbs to make long strokes with firm pressure from the heel up to the toes.

- One at a time, massage each toe, being sure to get in between toes as well. Give each toe a gentle tug to loosen the joint.

- Starting from the center of your heel, use your thumbs to press outward, and use your fingers to rub the tops of your foot at the same time.

- Gently rotate the foot in all directions, stretching your ankle.

- Repeat with your other foot.

Whether you give yourself a massage, ask your partner to help you, or go to the priciest spa in town, massage is one of those healing tools that will have a profound impact on how you feel and help give you the strength to make other healing choices and changes in your life.

Baths

When was the last time you treated yourself to a bath? Well, consider it an assignment! Shut the door, light a candle, and tell your family you're unreachable for the next half hour—it's for your health!

But before you dissolve into the warm water, be sure to add 2 cups of epsom salts and ½ cup aluminum-free baking soda to the water (skip the soap or bubbles). Why? Among other benefits:

- Epsom salts improve the ability of the body to use insulin, reducing the incidence or severity of diabetes.

- They flush toxins and heavy metals from the cells, easing muscle pain and helping the body to eliminate harmful substances.

- They relieve stress. Excess adrenaline and stress are believed to drain magnesium, a natural stress reliever, from the body. Magnesium is necessary for the body to bind adequate amounts of serotonin, a mood-elevating chemical within the brain that creates a feeling of wellbeing and relaxation.

- And they improve absorption of nutrients.

- Baking soda also helps draw out toxins from the body, too.

- It also keeps the blood at a healthy pH, whereby it is able to carry more oxygen so that the body can efficiently eliminate waste.

- Baking soda has also been found to optimize kidney function as well as chelate the body by removing heavy metals.

- Baths help raise your body temperature relieving your thyroid of doing all the work

- Baths can also help you sleep better. I recommend taking a bath 2 hours before bedtime.

So go ahead and lock the door and enjoy a bath!

Sauna

Saunas are another "luxurious" way to promote detoxification of your body. They need to be undertaken with care, but a sauna has a TON of benefits including:

- Skin rejuvenation.

- Enhanced sweating that gently and safely helps eliminate all heavy metals and toxic chemicals.

- Decongesting the internal organs and stimulating circulation.

- Inhibiting the sympathetic nervous system, enabling the body to relax, heal and regenerate itself much faster.

- Oxygenating and hydrating the cells and organs, and improving circulation.

And lots more!

See if your local gym, city recreation center, or health spa has a sauna that you can use. Sometimes even hotel spas will allow guests to use the facilities for a minimal cost.

When using the sauna, it's important to remember:

- Start with just 15–20 minutes. Some people really enjoy the sauna, but start slow to avoid side effects at first.

- Drink 8–16 ounces of pure water before you sauna.

- Wipe off your sweat with a small towel every few minutes. (That's where the nasties are!)

- Leave the sauna right away if you feel faint, if you stop sweating, if your face turns bright red, or if your heart starts to race. This could indicate overheating or heat stroke.

- Shower off after you sauna and use a very small amount of natural soap.

- You can safely use the sauna as little as once or twice a

week to start, up to as much as once or twice a day (check with your doctor first though.)

Give Yourself Some TLC:

How does it make you feel in your body to consider spending money on yourself for something like a professional massage? Does it make you feel anxious? Excited? Guilty? Where are those feelings coming from? Explore these questions in your journal.

Journaling

I hope you've been doing some of the journaling prompts in this book as you read along, but if you haven't, I'd love for you to consider adding journaling to your self-care routine, and using this book as a place to start.

The doctor who diagnosed me with Hashimoto's suggested journaling, and I balked. I didn't think I was a writer, and the thought of pouring my heart out on paper wasn't at all appealing. I had always hated to write, and would never have considered myself a good writer or even a writer at all but then my osteopath also recommended I begin to journal as a method for healing.

He suggested, a few years ago, that I enroll in the Write to Be You course by Rory Green. It was *life-changing*. Journaling changed the way I saw myself and the world.

Now, not only do I write, I've written multiple books and I am a regular contributor as a health expert for several publications! I am more confident, better able to work through conflicts and I relieve a lot of stress and challenging emotions through journaling. This is one of the best ways to not only manage stress but to find your voice.

In fact, medical studies have begun to find evidence of the health benefits of journaling—everything from reducing symptoms of chronic health problems (hello!) to reducing anxiety, depression, and stress.

Don't think...just write. You'll be amazed at what comes out and how it can help you heal.

Give Yourself Some TLC:

If you haven't been writing your answers to these prompts out on paper, consider this your invitation to start. Actually writing out your thoughts has a much greater impact than just thinking. Don't let your perfectionism take over, requiring that you find the perfect notebook, the perfect pen. In fact, you can download my free digital journal right here: **www.YourBestThyroidLife.com/journal**

Start now, today, with whatever supplies you have on hand and answer this question: How have you let your voice be silenced?

Meditation

I know lots of people are intimidated by meditation, but it doesn't have to be difficult—and you certainly don't have to have achieved enlightenment to try it!

Meditation has been shown to have all kinds of health benefits. Many practitioners believe that the root of all illness is in the mind, and when we clear our "mental pollution" the body is better able to heal itself.

From a physical perspective, stress greatly affects the adrenal glands, and that is directly related to the health of your thyroid. The adrenal glands secrete hormones (cortisol, epinephrine and norepinephrine) to regulate the stress response. When it comes to your thyroid, the ways in which our adrenal glands respond has far reaching consequences.

Beyond the obvious daily stressors in our lives, the adrenal glands pump out more stress hormones when your blood sugar isn't regulated, your gut is leaky, you have food sensitivities (such as gluten), toxins and infections are present, or you are inflamed and under an autoimmune attack — as is the case with Hashimoto's disease! You can't look at one without the other and adrenal stress is one of the most important components.

Adrenal stress creates a host of symptoms such as fatigue, headaches, insomnia, mood swings, sugar and caffeine cravings, irritability and dizziness. It also weakens your immune system, causes hormonal imbalances, promotes the autoimmune response and disrupts the interactions between the hypothalamus, pituitary and adrenal glands. This affects how you react to stress or trauma, your temperature, digestion, immune system, mood, libido and energy. In fact, weak adrenal glands can mimic symptoms of thyroid disease—whether you actually have thyroid disease or not!

Long story short: when our psyche and nervous systems are stressed, our body can't function at its optimal level, and it can't heal itself as easily or as well as it should. By meditating, we can relieve that stress and give our body the space and resources it needs to heal.

After I was finally able to move to California to meet up with my husband after the accident, I started to follow Deepak Chopra's blog. Prior to the accident, by chance, I had started researching about how the body can repair itself. It was an interest of mine to stay young, healthy and vibrant. I noticed after moving back to the Midwest from living in California and Italy that many of the people I had graduated high school with looked about 10 years older than me. They were eating the traditional SAD (Standard American Diet), not exercising, still smoking cigarettes and drinking loads (we were still young, after all!) The other thing I noticed is that since many people were overweight there, the idea of what health looked liked had shifted for many of my old friends.

Instead of seeing themselves as out of shape or unhealthy, I was the one often accused of being anorexic because I ate moderate portions of healthy food and maintained a fit physique. A healthy person was seen as too thin while a medically overweight person was viewed as "normal."

Because of my desire to stay away from this mentality and not jump on the slippery slope of unhealthy habits, I decided to learn about how one stays youthful in terms of health, fitness and healing. My first foray into this concept was reading Deepak Chopra's books, "Grow Younger Live Longer" and "Quantum Healing." I was fascinated by what I read in those books and signed up for Deepak's newsletter.

One day, I received a message from him about a contest the Chopra Center was holding to win a free yoga retreat at their center in Carlsbad, CA. The contest was to share something you were doing that was environmentally friendly. I read the email and had that gut intuition that I was going to win this contest.

We were in full wedding planning mode and had taken a number of steps to make our wedding, reception and favors environmentally friendly. So I entered the contest....and won! I had never won anything before. It was so exciting! And, it was the first time since the accident that I had felt that "knowing" feeling. That I had connected with my gut and intuition and understood on a core level that something good was about to happen.

What I won was a three-day yoga retreat! While thrilling, the bad news was that we had to pay for our hotel and some of our meals. We had just been hit by the truck. I had just lost my job...and we had no money. Through a series of happy coincidences, though, I found myself able to attend this retreat which changed my life forever.

As I was still reeling from PTSD, my husband dropped me off at Union Station in Los Angeles to hop on a train to Carlsbad. From the moment I got on the train, I felt a transformation take place. I was taking a step toward healing, I could feel it in my bones!

Riding along the pacific coast in a train is an amazing way to travel. It was a bright, sunny day and I enjoyed watching the waves crash as I made my way down the coast. After a blissful couple of hours, alone with my thoughts (miss those days — mamas don't get those enough!), I stepped off the train and hailed a cab.

Wouldn't you know it, the cab driver was from my home state of Indiana. I detected that Hoosier accent and we became fast friends. He and a lovely women I met at the retreat, ended up shuttling me back and forth from the hotel to the retreat all weekend.

This retreat was billed as a yoga retreat. I thought it would be great for my broken body and spirit as I learned how to connect with myself physically and emotionally again. I had been doing yoga since 2000 so this sounded like a great opportunity. What I wasn't prepared for though was the emphasis placed on meditation, morning and evening and while doing yoga.

I remember staring at the schedule thinking, "6:30 am meditation?!?!? What? Who's going to get up for that...and why?" But since I'd won this thing, I wanted to experience it all and I got my butt up early each morning and made my way down to the retreat center for morning meditation, breakfast and then a course in meditation, why it's important and what it does for your body and mind. It was TRANSFORMATIVE.

Never before had I been able to get my brain to shut up.

NEVER. It had never been quiet before. I'm a thinker and an analyzer and a chatterbox (both in my head and in real life – sorry friends!). Meditating three times a day changed the way my brain and I worked together. It allowed me to feel truly at peace for the first time in years.

Now, it wasn't without it's challenges. I'm no Zen monk. I certainly have monkey mind... but at that retreat, I learned techniques to turn down the noise in my head a bit. In one meditation session, I even saw colors. Trippy! And, pretty amazing. On the days I meditate and see colors, I really find a place of peace.

When you're ready to give meditation a try, you can use an app or MP3 to guide you, or just practice sitting and being. Yes, it'll feel weird and uncomfortable at first! We're not really used to sitting still with our thoughts. But like all things, it gets easier as you practice.

Start with just five minutes a day. You might choose to do it right when you wake up, or right before bed at night, but anytime, anywhere you can find five quiet minutes is the right time and place!

Try this:

- Sit in a quiet, peaceful environment at a time when you won't be disturbed. First thing in the morning is great, but any time you can find is perfect.

- Get rid of distractions. Turn off the TV. Silence your phone. Put on soothing music if you like.

- Find a comfortable place and position to sit. On the ground is great. Use cushions and pillows to make yourself comfortable. And if you can't sit on the floor, there's no reason you can't sit in a chair or even on your bed.

- Start with just 5 minutes a day. Set a timer. Try to work yourself up to 20 minutes per day.

- Close your eyes and focus on your breath. Try to just focus on breathing in and out.

- But when thoughts come (and they will!) release them without judgement. I like to picture a river and I set each thought in a little boat in the river and send it away.

Just like with any skill from catching a ball to playing the piano, you'll get better at this with time. It's likely you'll never be able to sit without *some* thoughts appearing, and that's OK! This is not about perfection, but rather about being present, about being here in this moment, and about practicing non-judgment and peace.

Give Yourself Some TLC:

What does peace mean to you? Describe a peaceful moment or place. What does peace look like in your daily life? How could you bring more peace into your life?

CHAPTER 8

Stress and Healing

PRIOR TO BECOMING hypothyroid, I could handle any stress… every stress really. Whatever came my way, I was able to deflect, like Wonder Woman with her magic bracelets.

Then I had my baby. After that, everything changed. I remember lying on the bed wanting to crawl out of my skin. As I stared up at the ceiling, waves of panic overtook me…but I wasn't sure why. I thought this was just hormones and the intense sleep deprivation of new motherhood.

Eventually, I learned it was my thyroid—powerful and completely out-of-whack.

As we now know, the adrenals, thyroid and our gut are inextricably linked. So it's a chicken and egg scenario as to whether a malfunctioning thyroid affects your adrenals or if your adrenals are taxed and that affects your thyroid.

When you're dealing with a health challenge such as a Hashimoto's disease, it's absolutely imperative to minimize stress and ask for help. I discovered that I need at least an hour a day to do something I enjoy, take care of myself and nurture my spirit, and that's what I recommend to all of my clients.

It was definitely a challenge to find the time for this. Remember: I had a toddler, a husband, a house, a life that needed caring for. But I realized that if any of those things were actually going to get taken care of, I had to take care of myself as well. I had to remind myself that it is *not* selfish to make any changes you need to support your health. Please remember that loving yourself comes in many different forms. This can be one of the hardest hurdles my clients tackle, but also one of the most important.

That's all well and good to say, but it takes real *work* to make that blissful me-time happen. I had to majorly shift my priorities and become a time management ninja.

For many people, these practices come in the cocoon phase of healing. Once you've made the major commitment to nourishing yourself back to health, it's important to take a look at how you can continue to support your healing process, and these important skills help you do that.

Honing my Ninja Time Management Skills

You know how it feels—you are greeted in the morning by a thick blanket of fatigue. You hardly want to lift your body up to get out of bed, let alone address the day's commitments.

When your body goes haywire due to a thyroid imbalance, your world gets turned upside down. The simplest task feels impossible to do so you start hiding from your "to-do's" and you pare your schedule down a bit.

And then the guilt comes in. You're not doing all that was once expected of you. You feel like a failure in your career, as a spouse, a friend or as a parent.

Here's the problem though....guilt physiologically creates a boat load of stress for your body. It creates anxiety in the mind which, in turn, creates stress in your system. You don't need to feel guilty. What you do need to do is heal! So please stop feeling guilty.

Now is not the time to be a superhero. Now is the time to redesign your life for optimal healing. Once you're healed, you can go back to leaping tall buildings in a single bound (if you actually want to). For now, you need to release yourself from guilt and ask for the help you need.

Maybe you didn't realize this, but so often we *continue* to attack our adrenals and ourselves by actually accepting stress into our lives. "Accept stress into my life," you wonder? "But I don't accept stress. Stress just finds me. It surrounds me...."

After I became I coach, I started to hear that a LOT — and it was something I used to believe, too. But what I realized is that most of the time, stress is a choice, and if you're feeling stressed, you've probably invited those stressors in, whether you knew it or not.

Here are some ways we accept stress into our lives:

1. We let other people's problems become our problems

2. We insist on doing everything ourselves

3. We let other people dictate our schedule

4. We feel guilty that we're "not doing enough"

5. We don't ask for the support that we need.

Other people's problems are NOT yours. Their "emergencies" are NOT for you to solve. You have plenty on your plate to deal with right now.

You need to create some healthy, loving boundaries, because right now is not the time to take on others' problems. You need to carve out time for yourself. Right now, you're the one who needs support.

Just like many women with Hashimoto's, I am a Type-A go-getter. I cram about a zillion things into my day and now finally, some of them are actually good for me! I went from all work and no play to carving out a 4-hour stretch, once a week, that's just for my self-care — that could mean a massage, journaling by the ocean, browsing at Anthropologie sans hubby and kid or just sitting alone someplace beautiful people watching. I give myself this gift every week and make sure to schedule in at least 1 nourishing thing a day to keep me on track. Learning how to manage my time with the right things has made me more efficient and my life more grounded, balanced and enjoyable.

One of the first exercises I do with my clients is to take a step back, breathe, and look at their schedule. I present them with a blank schedule and have them fill out everything they do on a given day on the first schedule. Then we go over it with a fine tooth comb.

I ask over and over again, "Is this essential? Do YOU have to be the one to do this?"

We love to think of ourselves as indispensable — especially we women and moms. We have this vision that if we don't handle everything, *nothing* will get handled. But the truth is, we need to give our partners, our kids, our friends and family a little more credit.

At some point, I had to admit that I didn't have to be the one to scrub the toilets in my house. SHOCKING, I know! But it came to the point that hiring a house cleaner was the right decision to make for my health, my relationship with my husband, and our sanity.

Of course, there was a whisper from that Midwestern girl in me that said, "This is crazy! You don't have money for a house cleaner. You don't even have a job!"

And I had to gently but firmly tell that voice to take a hike. This wasn't a luxury for us at that time; this was an all-out necessity if I wanted to heal (and we didn't want to live in filth in the process).

And now we *love* working with a house cleaner. I can't imagine my life without her!

As you start becoming a time-management ninja, you and your partner or family members may all have to take a hard look at your commitments and see where you are losing time, how you can be more efficient, and what kind of support you need to ask for.

- Can one or both of you ask your boss if you can work from home a few days a week?

- Can one of you run all the errands on one day instead of driving back and forth all week?

- What areas in your life can you tweak your schedule so that you are in control of it instead of the other way around?

- Where are the redundancies in the week?

- Where can things be done more efficiently?

- Where are areas you can find support? (e.g.—Can someone else pick up your kids once or twice a week so you can go to the gym or workout uninterrupted at home?)

Any time a new commitment comes up or someone needs help, ask yourself, "Will the world explode if I don't do this? Do I really need to do this now?" You'd be surprised at how many things you don't really need to participate in. Be firm with anyone trying to suck your time. Tell them that right now you have to take time to honor your health and cannot take on any commitments at this time. Be the guardian of your schedule and STAY FIRM.

I know: you've got a job, you've got kids or you've got a host of outside commitments. What's left for taking care of yourself— or your loved one? Well, unfortunately, in this society, no one is going to hand you a block of time. We don't live in a culture of daily siestas. We have to actually make a decision to take control and carve out time for ourselves.

When we're over scheduled and running on adrenaline, we tax our bodies and create more stress. How do you get a handle on it all? You empower yourself by realizing that this is YOUR life and you need to design it for yourself. Yes, there are obligations that can't be avoided but there are ways to redefine your schedule to promote overall health and wellness.

Real Life TLC Success:
Tamara, Age 37, Mother of 2, Professional

Tamara came to me after a frightening trip to the doctor's office where she learned she had low level antibodies (borderline) for several autoimmune disorders. She also was diagnosed with a fatty liver, pre-diabetes and stress-induced early menopause. She was 35 pounds overweight and felt overwhelmed with her health and lack of work/life balance.

Tamara was referred to me by her doctor who believed she needed to make significant changes in her diet and lifestyle. We worked together over the next few months to improve her overall health and stress levels.

Tamara's struggle was really about time management.

Juggling a career and two small children made it challenging for Tamara to find time for self-care and meal prep. So, we first looked at her schedule and found opportunities where she could get support from her husband, in-laws and her parents (the support team.) Then we laid out who could be in charge of carpool, meal prep and child care, whether it was Tamara or her support team, each day so that she could fit time in for daily exercise and self-care.

Next we looked at the family menu plan. With a household of picky eaters and children showing some behavioral challenges, we chose a meal plan that would both allow her to heal, help the children and be so delicious that the entire house would enjoy. We chose meals that could be prepped in 20 minutes or less and simple enough that anyone on her support team could prepare. We devised a prep plan that showed exactly what to prepare and when so that meal times were stress-free and joyful occasions.

Tamara lost 22 lbs in the first 6-weeks we worked together and the rest of the weight by the end of her program. By using a systematic approach to creating a personal and family schedule that minimized her stress level, and empowering and encouraging her to stick to the plan, Tamara was able to make impactful changes.

She now exercises consistently every day, eats and prepares nourishing meals, has reduced her stress, reversed the autoimmune response, pre-menopausal and pre-diabetic conditions and maintained a healthy weight that keeps her energized throughout the day. And, I received a lovely note from her doctor who was thrilled with her progress!

Techniques for Managing Your Stress

Figuring out how to eliminate stressors from your life is extremely important, but let's face it: you can't get rid of *everything* in your life that might possibly cause you stress, nor would you want to. You may work outside the home, have kids, drive in traffic, or heck pay taxes! And any one of those things can make you feel stressed, anxious or panicky from time to time.

But what we do have to do is take steps to alleviate that stress and anxiety when it does happen. In the last chapter, I talked about self-care, and stress reduction is a big part of that. Massage, journaling, and meditation have all helped me reduce my stress load, but why stop there? Here are some tips to manage stress when it arises.

1. Breathe

You knew this one would be first! But it's true, you've got to stop yourself and start breathing. If you do one thing, it's this... take a moment to breathe. Panic attacks can be accompanied by hyperventilation. So, it's important to focus on breathing slowly. Thyroid imbalances, anxiety and panic attacks can go hand in hand. It's important to head them off at the pass.

I love Dr. Andrew Weil's Breathing Technique. I use it whenever I can remember to but if I don't remember, I always go to my standby—taking a deep breath for 5 counts, holding for 3 counts and exhaling for as long as I can. Then I repeat. Deep breathing changes things on a physiological level.

If you can't slow your breathing down, it's time to get the ol' paper bag out to slow your breathing. Hold it over your mouth and progressively start slowing your breath so you can begin deep breathing. You'll want to do this for several minutes until you notice yourself calming down and coming back to earth.

2. Support your adrenals with food

There are many things you can do to support your adrenals through diet — and the things we talked about in earlier in the book are a great place to start! But you may need to talk to a health coach, functional doctor, or nutritionist to build a plan that's right for you.

3. Flex your muscles

A wonderful technique for easing yourself during a high-stress time or panic attack is to use progressive muscle relaxation. This not only helps you concentrate so you can slow your breathing, it diverts your attention from the trigger and helps your muscles relax. What you do is go from head to toe, starting with the muscles in your face, then on to your arms, hands, stomach, yo' booty, thighs, calves and feet. You'll tense each muscle group for 10 seconds and then release.

4. Smile, laugh and have fun

If you're at home when you start freaking out, I highly recommend throwing on your favorite funny movie. The act of cueing up the movie will require focus that will help you calm down. The laughter that comes from it will release happy hormones to help you get out of your head and back in your smile. If that doesn't work, call your inappropriate friend or colleague and have them dish out something funny—you know they will.

5. Try Holy Basil

Holy Basil, or tulsi as it is also known, is a plant used in Ayurvedic medicine as an adaptogen to modulate the stress response and support the adrenals. You can find tinctures of Holy Basil at health food stores, homeopathic pharmacies and some grocery stores including Whole Foods. Holy Basil is a potent herb so you'll want to try a few drops in a small glass of water first to see how it goes and use up to the maximum amount suggested on the bottle if it is well tolerated. I use it for stress and as a sleep aid when necessary.

Panax ginseng, Siberian ginseng and Ashwagandha can be used as well but should be taken only under the supervision of an experienced herbalist or trained practitioner.

6. Write it out!

One of the best things I ever did to help reverse this godforsaken disease is to learn how to write. When anxiety creeps in, start writing. You can grab any ol' piece of paper, keep a "panic diary" or use your journal. Acknowledge your anxiety and write out how you are feeling, what you are afraid of what you believe is triggering the stress.

7. Push the "panic button" on your stereo.

Turn that bad boy on—it's time to sing and dance out the crazy talk in your head! Now this can go two ways—you can put on your favorite relaxation playlist or you can put on those songs that make you wanna belt it out and shake your booty. Either way, you'll be doing yourself a great favor. Music has been shown time and time again to positively affect moods and reduce stress. You'll know when the mood is ripe to choose this option to chill.

8. Use aromatherapy

Fragrances can have a physiological effect on our moods. Burning incense, lighting a candle or using calming essential oils like lavender or chamomile or grounding essential oils that are spicy and earthy can calm our bodies (slowing heart rate, lowering blood pressure and relaxing muscles). You can mix some lavender drops (or other essential oils) and water and spray on a handkerchief. Lie down and place the handkerchief over your eyes as you rest and focus on your breath. It's a winning combination.

9. Calgon, take me away! (us old folks remember that)

This is my go-to get over it panic attack remedy. Pour 2 cups of Epsom Salts in a warm bath and get in. This will raise magnesium levels in your body and will have a calming effect on your mind by relaxing the nervous system, lowering cortisol levels and reducing the excitability of the brain. It works EVERY time! And hey, throw a little of that lavender oil in there for some extra relax in your remedy.

10. **Take a virtual vacation.**

Using guided imagery can be extremely effective in putting the kibosh on panic. Just think of a place or situation in which you feel completely at peace and relaxed. Close your eyes and imagine this place in detail. What does it look like? Who's with you (if anyone?) What are the sights, sounds and scents surrounding you? Paint a vivid picture in your mind and focus on it. When you notice your breathing and your body relaxing, you can open your eyes.

Don't let your desire to reduce stress actually create more stress to you and your nervous system. The best thing you can do is to relax about it all. Be aware but be relaxed. You have your tools now. When stress arises, talk to it, give it a little wave and let it pass you by.

Give Yourself Some TLC:

What are your best stress-busting techniques? Make a list of things that help you in your journal.

When You Can't Breathe:
Dealing with Overwhelming Emotions

She looked down and smiled at me, "We just can't get you to breathe, can we?" Yaffa, my new Pilates instructor, has only known me for two weeks. And since she has known me, Yaffa has probably had to remind me a few hundred times to exhale. I'm literally not breathing.

This was after two weeks of massive production mode. I've continued creating videos and hosting expert Q&A calls, I've recorded more than 20 videos as a free thyroid resource, I've been juggling motherhood.....oh, and my friend took her own life only hours after I posted an article on suicide. (Please read it here if you need help: http://bit.ly/ThyroidDepression)

So, yeah, those two weeks felt like being punched in the face over and over again — hence the non-breathing.

Not only had I not been able to breathe though, I hadn't been able to cry either. Shocked by the devastating news that I'd lost a dear, sweet friend, I sat stunned, choked up, gasping and sobbing for about 90 seconds...and then it all went inside. Locked up in my throat with nowhere to go.

This happens to me when I'm overwhelmed by emotion, overcome by sadness, shocked into emptiness. I stop breathing.... And I don't even know how to cry.... I go numb.

I forget sometimes that as a coach, I'm still human. As a recovering Type-A perfectionist, I, like many of my dear clients, hold myself up to an impossible standard. I always put so much energy into caring for my family, friends and our wonderful thyroid community that sometimes I forget that I need support too.

After speaking with another health practitioner, I realized I was really sad and stressed. (Shocker, right? But sometimes we need an outside perspective.) The past two weeks of being on camera (which is WAY out of my comfort zone for this introvert) as well as experiencing a tragic loss was just too much; and it would have been too much for anyone.

I finally heard the sadness as I was telling my story. It had been buried in the distraction of a busy life and now it was starting to bubble up.

Speaking with my colleague, the feelings started to move; heading to Pilates afterward, Yaffa got me to breathe; but calling my friend Lisa, got me to cry.... and that was just what I needed.

Lisa is my crying buddy. She's really my emotional soul sister. Lisa and I have been through some severe life events together over the past (almost 20!) years, holding each other up time and time again.

When I finally let the breath into my being and I could feel that block of tightness and sadness break apart, I knew I needed to move it out of my body. It wasn't serving me at all to keep it stuck there. So, I called Lisa and said, "I'm calling you so I can cry," and I told her my story.

Saying out loud that I lost my friend opened the gateway to healing. Having a witness to your pain, someone there to hold the space as you move through it is an invaluable tool for healing.

We all face overwork, overwhelm and tragedies, but what do we do with them in our bodies and how can that affect our health?

How breathing and crying can help you heal:

Here's why it's important to breathe, to protect self-care time, to sit with your emotions and to find your cry buddy.

- If you find you're chronically busy, it may not be that you have so much to do, but that you're avoiding being still with your thoughts. While we do live in an overscheduled world, it is often too easy to distract ourselves with busyness or to numb ourselves with TV keeping us from facing the reality of our lives. A busy schedule can be used to distract ourselves from our true feelings, but if you keep busy for too long, it can hinder processing emotions. And while you can ignore unpleasant emotions for a while, they don't go away until you address them. Hiding behind your schedule is a way of hiding from your feelings, either because you're afraid of feeling them, afraid that the sadness or anger will overwhelm you or never end, or you're afraid of how others will react. But it's important to find a safe way to experience those feelings (like with a cry buddy — see below).

- My Pilates teacher wasn't just toeing the party line when

she told me to breathe: proper breathing is detoxifying, releases tension, strengthens the immune system, and can even help you lose weight — in addition to helping release and work through emotions. So, let's make a pact to just keep breathing!

- Loads of people are embarrassed to cry or think "big girls don't cry," but research consistently shows that people feel relief and release after a good cry. Crying slows your breathing, has a calming effect and reduces stress; all which promote healing both physically and emotionally. Hey, there's a reason it's referred to as a "good" cry.

- But crying alone may not be the best idea. People who have support while crying report more cathartic release than people who cry alone, whether they rely on a friend, a therapist, a health care practitioner, or a support group… It's also true that having a partner for accountability and support can help you reach your bigger health goals, whatever they may be. So buddy up!

I feel so grateful to have someone in my life I can call my cry buddy. Lisa and I have struck an unspoken agreement over the years that we can say and be anything with each other. We let it all hang loose! When we're on the phone or hanging out, we're like two drunken pirates talking most of the time. Our "colorful" language would make any man blush and we're each other's safe place to go to let it ALL out, to laugh irreverently and to sob uncontrollably with each other as we work through pain. A cry buddy is one of the most valuable treasures I have in my healing kit. I highly recommend you get one.

Give Yourself Some TLC:

Who is *your* cry buddy? Who can you turn to in times of need, no matter what? Make a note so you don't forget that you can call on him or her when you need to! And if you don't have one yet, put on your favorite tear jerking film. It'll work like a charm.

PART 3:

Freeing the Butterfly

CHAPTER 9

Building Your Healing Plan

NOW THAT YOU'RE ARMED with the information you need to nurture your body back to health, crafting your own healing plan will be a snap. Here are the steps to creating your own unique healing program:

1. Make a list of friends, family, colleagues, neighbors, etc. who you know would be willing to actively support you in kicking thyroid, autoimmune or inflammatory disease to the curb.

2. Next to his/her name, write out the ways they could (or you wish they would) help you.

3. Now create a Time Management Ninja spreadsheet. Write or type in the absolutely fixed "to-do's" in your life, like work, school, shuttling kids to practices, preparing nourishing food for yourself or your family.

4. Once those are in, take a moment to see if there are any opportunities for you to find support to free up some time. For instance, can you split carpool responsibilities

with someone or can a friend, family member or neighbor watch the kids so you can get time to journal, be in nature or exercise? Can you and your colleague take turns bringing in fresh, home-cooked meals or salads for each other for lunch? Can you and a neighbor or friend take turns hosting simple family dinners or pitch-ins so neither of you are responsible for getting dinner on the table every night. We're looking for opportunities to create larger pockets of time for self-care here so start noodling and get creative.

5. Now it's time to actually ask for help. Reach out to your friends, family, colleagues and neighbors. Tell them that you're tired of being in the grips of this depleting disease and ask if they will commit to supporting you for the next few months so you can get back to being your normal, happy, vibrant self. Then specifically let them know the different ways they could provide support. If you need help getting the conversation started, use the letter we gave you in Chapter 7 as your guide.

6. Next, list out all the techniques from this book that you'd like to continue to implement to support your healing. So, if you want to include time in your schedule for things like dry brushing, sauna, Epsom salt baths, massage, fitness, or anything else, type or write those into your schedule.

7. Make sure to carve out time each day for the following in your new healing schedule:

    •   Stress Reduction: 10 minutes for meditation/

breathing exercises

- Fitness: 30 minutes for light exercise

- Detox: 30 minutes for a daily Epsom salt bath or sauna

- Self-love: 10 minutes for writing in your journal

- Brain reboot: 10 minutes for a walk outside or around the office mid-day

- R & R: 30 minutes for something playful (doing a hobby, horsing around with your kids, dancing to your favorite music, watching a funny TV show, trading massages with your honey, something that will make you laugh and smile)

I'm asking you to commit to yourself for 2 out of 24 hours every day so you can feel better, have the energy to do all the things you want to do and be the friend, parent, partner, colleague, son/daughter you have been wanting to be.

8. If you're like me, my mind is in a million places and my schedule is generally fuller than I'd like. We live in a society that doesn't reward family or chill time like my beloved Italy. So, what I do to make sure I can actually remember to do all the wonderful things I want to do to support my health is to add alarms to my phone's calendar. I have a daily alarm for fitness, going outside, meditating, reading and journaling. I even have alarms that say, "practice Italian!" and "tap dance class" (yes, I'm

a nerd). This is so I remember to make the things that I LOVE to do a priority. Those all go on the schedule and get an alarm. Setting an alarm can bring you right back into the present moment with reminders of what's truly important to you so that you can remember to do those things for yourself instead of getting mired down by doing the bills, dishes, laundry or working around the clock. You owe it to yourself to make your health and happiness a priority.

9. And finally, seek out a health coach, functional doctor, and other practitioners to create a healing team. There isn't one practitioner who can do everything for you. Functional doctors are great for ordering and assessing lab work and suggesting the right medical and supplemental protocols for you. Health coaches are able to spend time between your medical appointments to craft a nutrition and lifestyle plan unique to you and your family's needs. They can also be your accountability partners to keep you on track.

What happens if I can't find the time to do everything I want to do?

First, review your schedule again and make sure that only mission critical to-dos are taking up the "fixed" part of your schedule (things like work). If something doesn't ABSOLUTELY have to be done and can be taken off the schedule, put it on hold for another time when you're feeling better and you can back down on your healing schedule a bit.

The other thing to consider is that you can add these new lifestyle techniques into your schedule a little more slowly. Add one thing at a time and as you heal, you can incorporate other healing techniques in its place. Remember though, the first things to cut out of your schedule are the non-essentials. Make sure you are truly obligated to a task before putting it before of your own self-care and healing.

Do you have to be at EVERY soccer practice, and if so, can you use that time to do some of your own fitness by walking around the field or track? Look for opportunities throughout your schedule to combine self-care activities with those "must-dos." You'll be amazed at what you can accomplish and you may just inspire others to do the same.

Check your attitude

Just in case there's a little voice in the back of your mind whispering that all this "body wisdom" and "heal yourself" talk is a little woo-woo, remember that the power of the mind in relation to healing is a proven fact.

Just believing that a treatment will work has incredible—and proven—benefits. It's called the placebo effect. And no, I'm not saying that what we're going to be doing here is the equivalent of sugar pills! What I'm saying is that Western medical science has documented the power of belief in healing over and over again.

How do you get your mind in tip-top shape for healing? In a great post, 6 Steps to Healing Yourself, on Zen Habits, (**http://zenhabits.net/heal/**) Lissa Rankin, MD, a leading alternative medicine practitioner, suggests six steps to get yourself in the mindset for healing:

1. Believe you can heal yourself. Really believe it.

2. Find the right support. That can include doctors, alternative medicine practitioners, and friends and family.

3. Listen to your body and your intuition. No one knows your body better than you do—no one! So whether it's advice from your doctor or something mentioned in this book, if it doesn't feel right, don't do it!

4. Diagnose the root causes of your illness. We're going to go through this step-by-step in the next section, but it's important to remember that your thyroid disease isn't just about your thyroid. It's about your body as a whole.

5. Write your own prescription. This doesn't mean medicine necessarily or even supplements, but rather a lifestyle prescription. We'll talk about this more in the next section.

6. Surrender attachment to a particular outcome. If you are really attached to a certain number of pounds or decreasing your medication to a certain dose, you may just miss the boat. Oftentimes, our healing comes to us in incremental steps forward. Hey, it took your body a long time to fall out of balance and it may take a while to get back to normal. Focusing all your attention on the

outcome (or goal) and not on the process can leave you defeated and feeling worse than before. Instead, focus on the journey (the victories, large and small) and not just the destination.

Resources — Best Books, Products & Online Support

In going through my own health journey with Hashimoto's, I did a *lot* of research, read a *lot* of books, and tried a whole *heckuva* lot of products in trying to figure out what worked best. That's awesome news for you, because I've done a lot of the leg work for you already! Check out all the free resources on my website ThyroidLovingCare.com to discover my favorite places for online support, books that will supplement this one and increase your understanding of your condition, products I use *daily* to support my healing, and tutorials I've produced to help get you on your way to health.

So, how do I get the support I need?

As I embarked on my healing journey, I built a healing team to help me achieve my health and lifestyle goals. My team included functional practitioners and doctors, a variety of coaches, energy workers and more. Throughout this process, I learned the best of what each had to offer, took additional training and became a health coach myself so I could support others with thyroid and autoimmune disease.

Imagine if you had the energy to do the things you wanted to do. Imagine if you were able to keep your weight to a healthy level without giving it much thought. Imagine if you had a partner advocating for you at the doctor, finding recipes that nourish you and fit in your schedule or help you get through a panic attack. What would life be like if you had all those things?

A health coach doesn't operate under the same strictures and demands as a primary care doctor. We can set our own schedules, spend as much time with a client as needed, and can brainstorm and implement solutions that go way beyond medicines and procedures. For chronic, lifestyle-related diseases (like thyroid and autoimmune disorders) a health coach can be much more effective at helping you develop specific regimens and goals that work with your life.

Lifestyle changes can be difficult to achieve. (We all know we should eat better and exercise, right?? But how many of us just do it?) Traditional doctors often don't have the time or the bandwidth to truly partner with their patients in achieving those changes just because of the way our medical system is set up.

Just like you might hire a personal trainer to help you navigate your new gym or reach a particular fitness goal, you can hire a health coach to help you navigate a complicated medical diagnosis and reach your health goals.

Coaching can mean the difference between healing being a pipe dream or your reality. To learn more about the very special, interactive coaching program and healing community I created to reverse symptoms and eliminate thyroid disease, I invite you to explore **ThyroidLovingCare.com**.

CHAPTER 10

Butterfly Rising:
How You Can Love Your Body
Back to Health

THE BUTTERFLY DOESN'T choose what she will become. Nature tells her what to do, and she goes through her metamorphosis — or withers. There is no other choice.

You, on the other hand, are blessed with free will. You get to make the choices that will carry you on to the next phase of your life... Or leave you stuck and unhappy. But either way, the choice is up to you.

Through years of disease and suffering, the process of making new choices to heal myself, and my reemergence as a health coach to help others through their transformations, I've come to realize one very important fact:

The small choices we make every day add up.

They add up to health — or disease. To happiness — or depression and confusion. To love — or self-flagellation.

And even when you think you're not doing anything, when you're not taking action, you're still making a choice.

You're choosing to stay stuck.

Health is all about *choices*:

Choosing herbal tea over coffee.

Choosing gluten-free pasta instead of traditional pasta.

Choosing nuts and seeds for a snack over a candy bar.

Choosing water over soda.

Choosing 15 minutes of exercise instead of another hour of watching TV.

What do you choose to become today?

I choose peaceful, vibrant and healthy. Every day, we are faced with a choice. We can choose to do the things that nourish us or those that don't.

It is always easy to come up with an excuse as to why we can't do this or that....why we can't find time to take care of ourselves... why we don't have the time or energy to cook for ourselves or eat real food. We can easily find excuses. But those excuses are what's keeping you from healing. When you make choices that aren't nourishing, you're saying to yourself and the world that this donut, piece of cake, cookie, pizza, pasta, bag of chips, fast food, fast life, hustle and bustle is actually more important than you and your health. You're saying it's more important than your family... because an unhealthy you is an unhappy you and that's not what you or your family and friends need. You are saying to yourself that those things are more important than YOU...that you don't deserve health...but you do! You deserve feeling great again..like yourself again..."normal" again. And you're worth it!

What do you choose for yourself today? When you get in a frazzled space or go to grab a food that you know is not good for your body or your thyroid, pause. Take a moment and ask yourself, "am I making the nourishing choice?"

No. More. Excuses.

If you take away anything from this book, I hope you will take this: Now is the time to choose health. Now is the time to make one small choice toward healing that will have huge ripple effects over time.

The Time Is Now.

Today, choose YOU. Choose healing.

APPENDIX

Real Life TLC Successes (in their words)

Emmy, Age 26, Professional

How TLC Radically Changed My Life – Forever.

It was my 25th birthday. I was in a new patient consult with a primary care physician. My only intentions for the visit were to get a renewed prescription for my thyroid medication – All I wanted was my medication, nothing else. I hadn't been to the doctor in at least a year and hadn't had a thorough physical exam in much longer. As this new doctor reviewed my new patient forms and asked me questions about my medical history, she opened a door for me that I didn't expect. She didn't just write me a prescription. She told me that I was nearly obese and we needed to do some intervening if I wanted to avoid getting sicker.

Worst. Birthday. Ever.

I left that appointment crying. No, not just crying. Panicking. Scared. Alone.

I had been teeter tottering on the edge of denial in regards to my ever-declining health for a long time. I knew I had gained weight, but in that appointment I found out that I gained way more than I realized. I knew I was feeling sick, but I was far sicker than I was aware.

A follow up appointment after several blood labs told me that I was very sick. My doctor was straight with me. She said, "if you continue getting sicker you'll struggle with fertility and getting pregnant. You will continue to feel fatigued, confused, depressed, and anxious. You'll continue gaining weight, and feeling miserable. You won't just be pre-diabetic, you'll become diabetic. Your future doesn't look good." She explored putting me on several medications but I knew that wasn't what I wanted for myself.

I became immediately overwhelmed. Where do I begin? I was scared I had dug myself into a hole that I wouldn't be able to get out of. After a good week or two of crying and being extremely unsure of what I was going to do to get better, I mustered up a little bit of courage to begin looking for alternative answers.

I researched endlessly and finally found a program that was about to change the rest of my life - Jen's Radical TLC Solution home healing program.

"Another weight loss program," I initially thought. I wondered if it would be worth it. I was afraid of being disappointed by another promised answer to good health. But I went for it, and what happened to me was far beyond my expectations.

* * *

7 Ways That TLC Radically Changed my Life

1. Weight loss

Before this program, I had a long history of working myself into the ground at the gym (with and without assistance of personal trainers). I tried SO many diets and even became Vegan for three years thinking that animal products were to blame. I tried everything in my power to figure out my body and what it needed to get healthy – nothing worked. I would just keep gaining.

After starting the program, I immediately lost ten pounds. And then ten more. And then ten MORE! 8 Months into the program, I've lost 35 pounds through diet and lifestyle changes alone. And let me tell you, 35 pounds has meant a lot to my tiny 5 foot body.

2. GERD Symptoms Vanished

Before this program, I'd have spells where I'd wake up in the middle of the night and need to vomit. I'd wake up in the morning, almost every day, feeling extremely nauseous. I'd have the worst acid reflux after eating and, eventually, eating became a source of anxiety for me. I couldn't pinpoint the foods that were causing me to feel this way. Doctors only encouraged me to take medication, which I refused to do.

After starting the program, it became immediately apparent to me which foods were causing this much digestive distress. All of these symptoms vanished within the first couple of weeks of the TLC protocol. No more vomiting, no more nausea, and no more food anxiety.

3. Body Pain Gone

Before TLC, my body hurt. All. The. Time. I made the classic old lady sounds when I'd stand up, lay down, sit down – well – okay pretty much all day, I sounded like an arthritic elderly woman when I moved.

After several weeks into the program, the pain went bye-bye. I was able to move in ways and for periods of times that I hadn't been able to in so long. This made my quality of life go up exponentially.

4. Improved Fatigue and Sleep

Before I found this program, I slept all the time. Anywhere from 10-14 hours at night, with a much needed nap in the afternoons or after work. Sometimes I would wake up on the weekend only to eat lunch and would immediately fall back asleep when I was finished. I would bounce back and forth from being able to sleep completely through the night to not being able to sleep a wink. This affected me immensely. People told me every day how tired I looked. I would get asked, often, if I was sick or feeling well, at the very appearance of my face. My eyes were swollen and puffy constantly. I was pale. I felt like I was living with a constant hangover and this made me extremely self-conscious. I was calling out sick from work, a lot.

After TLC, I experienced…. Relief. That's the best way to describe it. While I still struggle with crawling out of bed some mornings, it's far easier than it ever was prior to this program. I can get a solid 8 hours of sleep and get out of bed without feeling like I need to call in sick. I no longer rely on caffeine to get myself to function properly. I can sleep through the night, and rarely have a night where I can't. This has been one of my favorite parts of the program. Lack of sleep and quality rest is extremely hard on the body, I didn't quite realize this fully until I started healing.

5. Brain Fog Eliminated

You know that feeling when you walk into a room and immediately forget what you were going to do? That was my life all day, every day before this program. I had an extremely difficult time remembering small, easy details. I'd forget things very easily if I didn't write them down. Daily confusion and general brain fog was probably one of the most difficult parts of my life before the program.

After TLC, the fog cleared. I was able to get tasks done at work and at home with so much ease. As a public speaker, I was able to improve my presentations and speak to audiences in a very comfortable and confident way. I no longer need to pause in the middle of explaining something to remember what my point was. Needless to say, my work ethic has much improved.

6. My Skin Cleared Up

Hormonal Acne, anyone? My goodness. Before I got started with TLC, the acne along my jawline was awful. I was constantly breaking out with painful acne.

After TLC, my acne cleared up. My skin is smoother, vibrant and youthful. I love looking at my skin.

7. I Don't Feel Alone Anymore

Before I found The Radical TLC program, I didn't talk about my chronic health problems. Ever. It was information that I had and knew in the back of my head that I rarely ever disclosed to anyone. I suffered at work and in my personal life, but no one knew why.

An incredible perk of joining TLC, is the community that comes with it. Having other women to talk to about the suffering that comes along with chronic health problems, has been phenomenal in my own process to emotionally heal from everything I've been through. I talk to my husband regularly about how I'm feeling, emotionally and physically. I'm more connected to myself and to those around me because of it. I can openly share my story and my progress, because of this community.

* * *

You may be wondering if The Radical TLC approach to healing is for you. You may be questioning if this is the answer to your problems, just as I did. You may be telling yourself that it's not your diet, it's not your lifestyle, that it's something unknown to you at this present moment – and that all may be true. I certainly relate to all of those feelings. But - what this program did for me was force me to truly take a bird's eye view of my life. My diet. My stress. My ability to practice Self Care and put myself first above all else.

At the start, I was desperate and willing to do anything to find the road to recovery. I never would have dreamed that the road I was looking for was this program and never, even for a second, have I wanted to stray from it. If it weren't for Jen Wittman's radical program, there's no doubt in my mind that I'd be that obese, diabetic, infertile woman that my doctor warned me about 8 months ago. She gave me all the tools that I needed to save my life and I will never fully be able to express the gratitude I feel for her and her gift of health coaching. I couldn't have asked for more. – **Emmy**

Hannah, Age 33, Professional

"Having Lyme Disease, it has been really hard for me to take control of my health and do all the things I need to do to aid in my recovery process. Jen has taken that into her own hands and it has been an extreme load off of my plate and off of my mind. She did Lyme research for me, referred me to doctors that I would never have found on my own, she put me on a lyme friendly diet that has helped a lot of my symptoms ease up and she is always there to support me when I have questions and concerns.

I trust and take comfort in Jen's support because she has reversed her own autoimmune disorder by nutrition and self care. She understands what I am going through and how I feel and knows that I can get better, that in itself is mentally relieving to me as I have seen many, many doctors that have not taken me seriously and written me off while writing yet another prescription that did not work. Through my physical pain, fatigue and brain fog, I desperately needed someone to come in and give me stress relief techniques, Lyme facts and treatment options, continuous support and a nutrition plan and that is exactly what Jen did for me and so much more. It has been wonderful."

Katie, Age 29, Ph.D.

"Jen was instrumental in getting me through the last months of my Ph.D. with some semblance of a normal schedule. She provided tons of support on how to fit in everything I needed to do to get my degree while still keeping time for the things I needed to do for me like exercise or time with friends and family. Now that I'm through that push, she is helping me to develop a lifestyle and diet that's the healthiest for my body and to keep Lupus at bay."

Chad, 41, Business Owner

"Learning that some of my levels were creeping toward diabetes, I decided to undertake a sugar detox with Jen. I have to say it has changed my life. After 5 days I lost all cravings for sweets and starchy foods, with the exception of a few nighttime cravings. Those were easily overcome with the tools and tricks that Jen gave me to do so. I lost about a pound a day, totaling 20 lbs. I feel clearer, lighter and my daily aches and pains have reduced greatly. My jeans are baggy, and my shirts aren't tight anymore. I sometimes forget to eat, where before I was eating all of the time. But the best part is that my hunger has diminished so much, that I don't even finish my plate sometimes; and whatever I eat totally satisfies me! She's taught me about the importance of self-care, working through emotions and how it plays into cravings and healing. Working with Jen opened my eyes to stress & emotions I was storing in the body that was contributing to my ill-health. I am so grateful I had the opportunity to work with Jen to transform my life."

Acknowledgements

Thank you Lacy Boggs, my patient Editor, for bringing life to my words and sometimes disconnected thoughts. You have helped me lovingly articulate my mission, message and resources with the world that otherwise would not have seen the light of day.

Thank you to Rory Green for teaching me to love my words and to love to write. I could not have learned the meaning of my voice in a better way. Thank you for the gift of writing my truth, for empowering my healing and for introducing me to the most wonderful group of women, my Write To Be You sisters (Sophie, Helen, Jessica, Mady, Jennifer, Ami, Kim, and Jody).

Thank you Debbie Franco for giving me "Healing Foods" oh so many years ago which changed my life forever and set me on the path of using food to heal myself and others. You have been an ally through the roller coaster that has been my life for over a decade and I am grateful for your friendship.

Thank you to Rochelle Torke for helping me bring Thyroid Loving Care to life and for being my first spiritual teacher (even if you didn't know it).

Thank you to my parents (Cindi Gilbert & Chuck Wittman) and my sister, Allison Wittman for just being you, for just being there and for just being my family. I'm lucky that you're mine.

Thank you to Doug and Bodhi Sanders for loving and caring for me every. single. day.

Thank you to Elisa Calderon for being there over the years to care for our home. No one puts more love into their work than you. Thank you for helping me take care of Bodhi over the years and whenever we visit Los Angeles.

Thank you to everyone who makes up my family by blood or by choice and to my dear friends (I'm not listing you all out separately because inevitably, I'll forget someone and feel like a jerk! but you all know who you are). Thank you for standing by me when I'd fall asleep on my couch at my own party at 9 pm over and over again. Thank you for jumping in to watch Bodhi when I needed it, for taking me on dates with the understanding that I have to eat dinner when "blue hairs" and children do in order to feel my best, for wiping off my tears through the accident, the lawsuit, the losses and the illness, and for your willingness to provide your love and support, your encouragement and acceptance at every step of my healing journey.

Thank you to the doctors, practitioners and energy workers whose talent and caring have helped me forge my path in health and coaching. I truly appreciate all that you've shared and done for me.

And, finally, thank YOU, dear reader. You have just taken a wonderful step toward nourishing, caring and loving yourself. Your desire to thrive with thyroid disease makes you a hero in my book, literally. You're in my book and I'm calling you a hero right now. You are awesome and you will feel like yourself again soon, I just know it!

References

Rankin, Lissa, M.D. 2013. 6 Steps To Healing Yourself.
ZenHabits.net/heal

Kresser, Chris, M.S., L.Ac. 2014. Thyroid Disorders.

Medical Disclaimer

The information provided in this book is designed to provide helpful information on the topics discussed. This book is not meant to be used, nor should it be used, to diagnose or treat any medical condition. This book is not intended as a substitute for the medical advice of physicians. The reader should regularly consult a physician in matters relating to his/her health and particularly with respect to any symptoms that may require diagnosis or medical attention.

The publisher and author are not responsible for any specific health or allergy needs that may require medical supervision and are not liable for any damages or negative consequences from any treatment, action, application or preparation, to any person reading or following the information in this book. References are provided for informational purposes only and do not constitute endorsement of any websites or other sources. Readers should be aware that the websites listed in this book may change.

22386363R00111

Made in the USA
Middletown, DE
29 July 2015